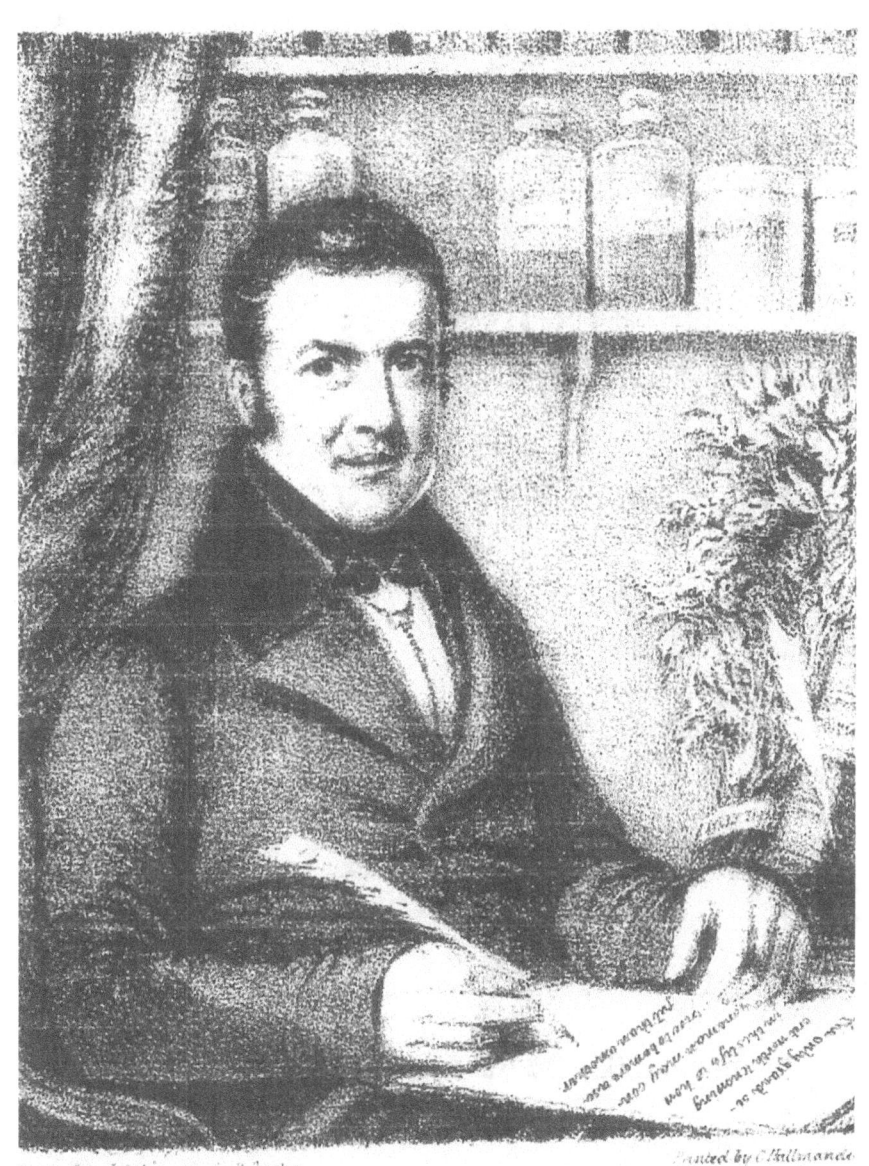

Drawn from Life & on stone by T. Denton.

Printed by C. Hullmandel.

Mᵣ S . W . TILKE .

Practical Botanist

Born at Sidmouth, Devon, 9ᵗʰ June 1794.

This Plate is presented to the Author by a grateful Patient

RANDOM REFLECTIONS

ON

INDIGESTION,
BILIOUS COMPLAINTS, SCOFULA &C.

BY   SAMUEL   WESTCOTT   TILKE,

MEDICAL HERBALIST.

2022 Transcription by J S Tilke

Published in 2023 by the transcriber, John Stuart Tilke

Tilke, Stuart
Random Reflections by Samuel Westcott Tilke,   2022 Transcription
ISBN: 9781447518846
        Imprint: Lulu.com

Autobiography/ Herbalism/ Botanical/ Victorian/ Sidmouth/ London/ Devon/ Medical/ Botanist/ Gout/ Scrofula/ Tic Devereux/ Digestion/ Ringworm/ Scarlet Fever/ Scald Head/ Dropsy/ Medical Profession

RANDOM REFLECTIONS

ON

INDIGESTION,
BILIOUS COMPLAINTS, SCROFULA, &c.

OBSERVATIONS
ON THE
NATURE AND CURE OF GOUT.

REMARKS
ON
DISEASES OF THE SCALP,
INCLUDING THE
RING - WORM.

AND SUGGESTIONS ON THE TREATMENT
OF THE
SCARLET FEVER.

By S. W. TILKE.

" And the Lord God planted a garden in Eden: and there He put the man whom He had formed. And out of the ground made the Lord God to grow every tree that is pleasant to the sight, and good. " -- Gen. ii. 8, 9.
"And the fruit thereof shall be for meat, and the leaf thereof for medicine." -Ezek. xlvii. 12.

LONDON:

PRINTED BY J. POULTER, GT. CHESTERFIELD STREET.

1837

1568 / 6665.

" I pray thee understand a plain man,

In his plain meaning."

SHAKSPEARE.

PREFACE

TO THE THIRD EDITION.

"Men should be what they seem;
Or those that are not, would they might seem knaves. "

"I have neither the scholar's melancholy, which is emulation;
nor the musician's, which is fantastical; nor the courtier's, which
is proud; nor the soldier's, which is ambitious; nor the lawyer's,
which is politic; nor the lady's, which is nice; nor the lover's,
which is all these. But it is a melancholy of mine own;
compounded of many simples, extracted from many objects; and,
indeed, the sundry contemplation of my studies, in which my
often rumination wraps me in a most humorous sadness." - SHAKSPEARE.

While I was yet in doubt whether I should find it necessary to burthen my readers with a Preface to this, my Third Edition, I had put into my hands a newspaper, giving an account of a meeting held at Exeter Hall in December 1836, which I cannot do better than introduce here, that my readers may see how anxious *"the profession"* are to put fetters on those who do not, like themselves, possess *diplomas,* to shield them from the consequences of their own acts. "

The following is copied *verbatim,* as I will

"Nothing extenuate
Nor set down aught in malice." - SHAKSPEARE.

"MEDICAL EXPOSURES. - *Meeting at Exeter Hall— The immaculate Colleges —Wretched State of the Profession - The new Pharmacopœia, its Blunders and gross Prejudices.*

"On the 19th of December 1836, there was held, at Exeter Hall, a meeting of the British Medical Association; and if any one circumstance more than another could have opened the eyes of the public to the enormities of Medical Practice, it must have been that meeting. We naturally look to the *schools* of any particular science for an illustration of its worth: and the pupils emanating from these seminaries are certainly best qualified to describe their fitness. The College of Physicians, *par consequent,* is shown up by the British Medical Associates as only less infamous than the College of Surgeons. The latter is distinctly stated to be 'the most illiberal corporation in the kingdom;' the council grossly corrupt, and self-elected for life; and *apostacy* the only sure means to obtain reward! 'And can this state of things,' says the address, 'continue to exist much longer?' We opine *not;* and shall spare no efforts of our own to complete its utter extinction. At the meeting to which we have alluded, a worthy of the name of Murray, an M.D., made the following speech :-

"I beg to ask, Sir, is it your intention to obtain petitions to Parliament for protection against the monopolists of your own body on the one hand, and ignorant quacks and empirics on the other- from him who pours thousands of drastic pills down the throats of the people for every kind of disease, or to him who kills *after another fashion*!

"After what fashion! why, the fashion of the *M.D.s,* to be sure: and how does the reader suppose that Dr. Murray proposes to 'obviate deception' in like matters? Why, by 'legislative enactment!'. This is too good. The doctor would be the very man to regulate by Act of Parliament the number of potatoes we ought to swallow at a meal! The address comes much nearer the truth in speaking of the degraded state of the profession. 'The medical profession in this country has long been, and is at present, in a most unsettled and unsatisfactory state, whether we regard the position of the physician and the consulting surgeon, or that of the general practitioner. This has arisen *chiefly* from the *apathy*, the *jealousy*, and the *disunion* existing in the general body.' When *all* are corrupt-colleges, branches, and the individual members of an art to which that 'precious jewel', our health, is referred, - there is hope, at least, of being very securely put out of the way, and rid of the troubles of this life! In the face of so much obloquy, one would fancy that the mighty 'Pharmacopoeia' of the College of Physicians would not have been put forth without a revision so stern as to defy the detection of error. No such thing: their *Parvum in Multo*, both in the original and translation, is rife of errors which professional men scruple not to call 'monstrous!' It appears as though it were reserved for the councils of colleges to do foolish things. They can recommend to Government the purchase of Mrs. Stevens' Stone -solvent, which turns out to be neither more nor less than soap-suds; and yet they can sit in conclave till midnight and decide not to in quire into the components of a medicine which Bransby Cooper and others have declared to be most unequivocally curative for its special purposes. Oh no! They decide *not* to send to Mr. Surgeon Franks, Blackfriars -road, because, forsooth, he has the protection of a patent; and yet Drs. Cholmondeley and Laird were always in the habit of sending to Newberry's for 'James' Fever Powders,' a patent medicine, until the secret of its composition was purchased by the *College* for two thousand pounds. The bitterest sarcasm ever dealt against the profession is self-inflicted, and consists in their denunciation of certain medicines of which they have not the skill to detect the ingredients, and effect cures in cases where *they* (the College-recognised ignoramuses) utterly fail!

"I.C."

This is what I foretold four years ago in my Second Edition (page 7 and 8). They now begin to feel, that "such men as myself would run away with all the meat; " or, rather, "with all their guineas;" I could give them another friendly hint, and say to them,

"I entreat you take no notice, nor build yourself a trouble
Out of this scattering and unsure observance,
It were not for your quiet, nor your good,
Nor for my manhood, honesty, or
Wisdom, to let you know my thoughts; " -
"But it is no matter,
Let Hercules himself do what he may,
The cat will mew, the dog will have his day."
SHAKSPEARE.

I have long wished for a parliamentary inquiry into the "MONOPOLY of the REGULARS on the one hand, and the IGNORANT QUACKS and EMPIRICS on the other:" each class being diametrically opposed to the public weal.

Should a Committee of the House of Commons be ordered to investigate this most important subject, I should rejoice in the opportunity of appearing before them; for I well know I could " a tale unfold," and show them with what comparative ease each of the rising generation might, (by introducing in our schools certain class-books and medical catechisms, prepared expressly to instruct the inquiring mind in the virtues of Nature's productions,) be most easily taught how to judge of their own constitutions, and to communicate the benefits of this knowledge to those who have not the same opportunity.

This would be the way to destroy all existing abuses, and effectually stop the nefarious proceedings of both the *legal* and *illegal* QUACK.

" For such things in false disloyal knaves
Are tricks of custom ; but in a man that's just
They are close denotements working from the
Heart, that passion cannot rule."- SHAKSPEARE.

The public might, with little effort, but good system, be speedily enabled to judge in a great measure for themselves, were such initiatory school- books on this particular subject brought forth, and which, if I can find the time, I fully intend to publish; wherein I shall shew the order and connection of natural things, together with the means whereby they are completed; I shall teach the youth how he may soon be conversant with the moral characters of men, and to attain a knowledge of all the arts (which are but the imitations of nature), with the advantages they provide for the welfare of man. I shall shew there is only one great book for them to study, to make them perfect; viz. the great and infallible book of Nature, which will shew them her remedial powers are inexhaustible. I shall teach them that "time and kindness" claims a large share in the rebuilding of the body, which must not be hurried by the handy -work of the physician. I shall prove to them, that Nature alone knows best how to restore, or repair her own materials, I shall endeavour to convince them, that I have enjoyed some of the pleasantest hours of my life in this delightful study. Hours stolen from my domestic circle, from the fatigue of business, and from the *time for sleep*. Acting in pursuit of this principle, the blessings to be found in the vegetable kingdom must be put forth; and knowledge, built on the principles of universal good to wards each other, such as rational beings should practise in matters appertaining to life and health, must be spread, if we hope to see abuses destroyed. We look for honesty of dealing in commercial and legal affairs; and I can assure the Council of "RHUBARB HALL," that in the practice of medicine a mighty change is about to take place, and probably much sooner than they expect or wish. This reform may be procrastinated, but cannot be avoided. Let the Faculty look to the rapid advances making daily in the science of botanical knowledge — a study which I delight in supporting and advocating

At a meeting of Ladies and Gentlemen lately held at the Botanical Institution, John-street, Adelphi, a paper was read by Mr. Irving, containing many facts relating to the science, and the results of observations made by him in its pursuit in the neighbourhood of London. It appears there are about 1,500 species of plants found in Great Britain, of which about 1,000 may be obtained within a circle of twenty-five miles round the metropolis, Mr. Irving had himself found 670 different species within two miles of Hampstead, and 900 within the same distance of the town of Croydon. The neighbourhood of London is considered the richest in the kingdom in objects of botanical research; the inhabitants of this smoky city have thus every encouragement to pursue this delightful and healthy employment.

Many of the Jessamys who attended Exeter Hall meeting have had their own way for some years past, and gone on like so many blind horses in a mill! Government might with great advantage export a ship-load of those gentlemen to explore the bounties of nature in savage lands; even among the unenlightened Sons of Nature, will frequently be found more rationality than is to be met with in the medical schools of London. Look at the medical squabbles which have been reported in the *Times* and *Morning Herald* these three years past; and mark the conduct of those men, whom education ought to have taught better: at St. Thomas's and London Hospitals; and at this moment at the Charing-cross Hospital, where it seems the contention between them is, not who shall do the most good for the suffering patients, but which of them shall carry away the largest portion of the   "loaves and fishes!" They are by these means bringing about (quite unintentionally) that wholesome change in their order, which I trust I shall live to see; and most assuredly the eyes of those who have the power to force this change, are "upon their doings."

Has the practical knowledge of the present day exceeded that of Shakspeare's Apothecary in "Romeo and Juliet," or his Doctor in "Macbeth?" Decidedly not. And this alone proves that physical science had attained, full two hundred years ago, at least, the same perfection that it has now, All the writings of Shakspeare and Le Sage evince that they had not a very high opinion of the doctors of their day. What would they say, if now living, on taking up the new pharmacopæia, to find seventy-nine *old* medicines designated by seventy-nine *new* names? By such folly, many mistakes have been made in prescriptions, and the danger of these alterations must be manifest. An Act of Parliament is really required to prevent this subterfuge for their utter want of the knowledge of Nature's medicines! Can I, or any other man, point out in too broad a character, the danger that may accrue to our *deceived*, *physic* taking, and *suffering* race?

> "If it were done, when 'tis done, then ' twere well
> It were done quickly."   SHAKSPEARE.

If my readers turn to the *Lancet* of January 7, 1837, they will there see the danger of giving new names to so dangerous a poison as "hydrocyanic acid. " This report emanates from Middlesex Hospital! If such a blunder had been committed by me, those "popinjays" of the profession would have been in arms to crush me in such a manner, as no enlightened mind can contemplate without disgust.

I have this moment a Prospectus before me, for the erection of a hospital, drawn by several of my most influential patients, and in which they propose to introduce my system, as practised so successfully in my own establishment for the last six years. I will only add, that I should not be found wanting on this occasion, but that my gratuitous services would be freely given in aid of so important an object. It is well known that I am already deeply occupied; but I should rejoice in the selection of six or more persevering and well-educated young men,[1] whose heads were on the right way, with one working man who had a thorough practical knowledge of anatomy, to attend to surgical cases, to whom I would very speedily make familiar my mode of action; and I would venture my future reputation on the report which should appear of our success, during even the first twelve months; such a detail, indeed, as should gratify the subscribers, and put some of the older institutions to the blush.

[1] *A young medical friend has put in my hand the following statement of the manner in which several years of the most valuable period of his life have been dwindled away, in acquiring what is called a* **competent** *knowledge of his profession: -— "A five years' residence with an eminent anatomist-a cooping up in a large parochial London Infirmary, to learn Pharmacy - a hospital dressership of twelve months, under a Sir Charles Bell - a session or two at Edinburgh, to see how the medical world wagged — then a diploma from the College of Surgeons, and a subsequent drilling in the fenny parts of Cambridgeshire - three nights in the week without ' passing through the sheets;' and all this trouble and expense, amounting to many hundreds, incurred before a shilling could be returned."*

It is not wonderful that these men, after spending so much time and money in **qualifying**, *as they call it, should feel anxious to indemnify themselves by over-dosing their patients- it is naturally to be expected. But what a waste of time for young men! who might, under* **judicious instruction**, *be* *early brought into action for the benefit of the afflicted, and for their own support. The vice is in the system!*

To return to Dr. Murray's Exeter Hall tirade: -

"Faith, sir, save your threats;
The bug, which you would fright me with,
I seek, I tell you.   'Tis Rigour, and not Law."

"There hath been much to do on both
Sides and the nation holds it no sin,
To urge them on to controversy."

"- When two authorities are up,
Neither supreme, how soon confusion
May enter 'twixt the gap of both, and take
The one by the other! " - SHAKSPEARE.

"There has been much throwing about of brains."
                                        SHAKSPEARE.

He could not surely mean me, when he said, "Or to him who kills after another fashion." If he does,

"I plead NOT GUILTY: my integrity
Being counted falsehood, shall, as I express it,
Be so received. But thus, if powers divine
Behold our human actions (as they do),
I doubt not then, but innocence shall make
False accusation blush, and tyranny
Tremble at patience."   SHAKSPEARE,

I can tell the learned Doctor, without fear of contradiction, that for the last eight years, with an extensive practice, frequently in very dangerous cases, I have been invariably successful; and I HAVE NEVER LOST A PATIENT UP TO THE PRESENT MOMENT, although by far the greater number have come to me after they were tired out by "the Profession," or had been told they were INCURABLE!! Can Dr. Murray say as much?

"But there is, sir, an aiery of children, *little* men, that cry out on the top of question, and are most tyrannically clapped for it; these are now the fashion, that many, wearing rapiers, are afraid of goose-quills, and dare scarce come thither." - SHAKSPEARE.

I would recommend my friends to read a pamphlet by "Frederick Salmon, M.R.C.S.," "One of their own body, "On the Necessity of an Entire Change in the Constitution and Government of the Royal College of Surgeons." He says, "The present arbitrary, irresponsible, and exclusive power of the Council is subversive of science, and derogatory to the public good." This is a pretty candid admission, but the truth of it cannot be disputed.

"Oh, gentlemen, the time of life is short;
To spend that shortness basely were too long,
If life did ride upon a dial's point,

Still ending at the arrival of an hour." - SHAKSPEARE.

Many of my sincere friends, even now, wish me to go through the regular degrees, as it is called, to get a *diploma* to PROTECT me. My answer is, my protection is, in my hundreds of grateful patients, in a liberal , and, I hope soon, a self-protecting public; and, above all, it is in my own bosom.

"What stronger breastplate than a heart untainted?
Thrice is he arm'd that hath his quarrel just;
And he but naked, though wrapt up in steel,
Whose conscience with injustice is corrupted."
SHAKSPEARE.

We all know what would be the examination to be gone through previous to gaining a *diploma*. But I will merely remind my readers, that I passed a more formidable ordeal several years ago, when I was invited to wait on one of the highest Medical Boards now existing in this country, to explain to them my views upon the nature and cure of disease. It is with pride I reflect on the liberal and gentlemanly observations which were addressed to me by several members of that Board; and, on taking my departure, the whole of them (fourteen in number) expressed their wishes for my success, and that they approved of all my replies to their questions, and would be happy to forward my views. Having passed this examination of an hour, with such gratifying results, what need I fear (if I were inclined) of three Examiners at Apothecaries' Hall? But

"I would rather be a toad,
And live upon the vapours of a dungeon."

In conclusion, I will only add, that the fact of this work being, from first to last, a series of *"Random Reflections,"* is not so much my fault as my misfortune. They are put down hastily, as passing events suggest them to my mind, however unconnected they may appear when put into print. Indeed, it is not possible, under my present arrangements, that it should be otherwise, as I write but a few sentences, and am then called away to severe exercise, both of body and mind; when I return, the thread of my ideas has been broken , and the mind flies off to other subjects. It will be sufficient encouragement if my friends find here and there some things worth perusing; and the recipes I have inserted, I can safely say, if generally acted upon, would mitigate an immense aggregate of suffering:

Very little time can be spared by me, while I prepare all my own medicines, and administer every dose, and attend the baths to all my in-door patients. Many visit me daily for consultation, to say nothing of the numerous letters I receive from the country, describing, oft-times, very difficult cases, and requiring either to be received in my house, or that I would send them medicine and directions. This of itself is a most responsible and arduous duty; and yet I rejoice in all this, inasmuch as there is a pleasure in mitigating the sufferings of my fellow-creatures, far outweighing all pecuniary recompense; and as in this latter respect I have nothing to desire, if I wish to do more, **IT IS THAT MORE GOOD MAY BE DONE.**

CONTENTS

TO

RANDOM REFLECTIONS.

RANDOM REFLECTIONS

ON

INDIGESTION, BILIOUS COMPLAINTS,

&c . &c.

"There was a time when all the body's members
Rebelled against the stomach - thus accused it:
That only, like a gulf, it did remain
In the midst of the body, idle and unactive,
Still cupboarding the food, never bearing
Like labour with the rest; where the other instruments
Did see - and hear - devise - instruct - walk - feel
And mutually participate, -did minister
Unto the appetite, and affection common
Of the whole body. The Stomach answered:-
"True it is, my incorporate friends," quoth he,
"That I receive the general food at first,
Which you do live upon; and fit it is,
Because I am the storehouse, and the shop
Of the whole body. But, if you do remember,
I send it through the rivers of the blood,
Even to the kidneys, the heart, to the seat of the brain;
And through the cranks and outlets of the body.
The strongest nerves, and small inferior veins,
From me receive that natural support
Whereby they live - and though that all at once, you, my good friends,
Cannot see what I do deliver out to each,
Yet I can make my audit up that all
From me do back receive the flour of all
And leave me but the bran ,-What say you to it? "

SHAKSPEARE.

From the balance of power between the several intellectual faculties of man, common sense has been said to have resulted. So likewise, in the regular and equable performance of the separate functions of the body, originates good health. By the consistent action of every organ the general fabric of the body is preserved, towards the maintenance of which the circulation of the blood performs a most essential office; and it appears to be a law of nature, that, in proportion as the function of any particular part is material to the health of man, so any deviation from its healthful condition produces a corresponding serious effect. We cannot but notice on every organ of the body, that nature assists herself in various ways; and our duty is to watch and assist her, in order to mitigate human suffering.

It is far from my intention to claim any superiority over my fellow *man* in the curative *art* - on the contrary, I am free to confess, that my talents do not rise above mediocrity; yet it will not be denied, that moderate abilities, combined with persevering industry and application, when directed to one single object, are more likely to succeed (and oftener do succeed) than the most splendid talents, which aim to embrace the whole circle of science at once. I am of opinion, (and this I speak from experience,) that every practitioner ought to spend much time by his patients' bed-side; thereby, with an observing mind, he may often gain a more practical knowledge than that gained in medical schools, or than the best medical works teach. By a diligent attendance on the sick, he may learn and fully understand the intimate connexion which subsists between the various parts of the human body - their mutual dependance on each other — their particular functions and uses; and how these are liable to be deranged by disease or other injury. These reflections will add fresh links to the chain of knowledge before attained , and ultimately lead to the accumulation of every truth that can throw new light on the disorder under his consideration. Here also, by diligent inquiry, he will ascertain, that by far the greater number of human maladies are curable by few and simple remedies, which are plentifully spread by the bounteous Author of Nature over the face of our island; such as will successfully oppose and compel a hasty retreat to many disorders, which have proved fatal to thousands of our countrymen - because too long deemed incurable. A patient, weakened both in body and mind, can do little towards the expulsion of an internal foe - unless nature be assisted in her constitutional efforts, by cordial, yet powerfully invigorating means, both by medicine and diet, which latter should contain a large quantity of nutriment in a small compass; instead of a starving debilitating system; such means will do infinitely more towards the restoration of health than drug enamoured persons may easily believe, or drug retailers be willing to allow.

> "There is scarce
> Honesty enough alive to make societies secure,
> But security enough to make fellowship unhappy;
> Much upon this riddle runs the world;
> This news is old enough, yet it is every day's news."
>   SHAKSPEARE.

Shakspeare has written -

> "There is no art
> To find the mind's construction in the face. "

On this principle, I think the ideas of an author ought to be poured out in such a simple manner as to be at once stamped on the mind of the reader; every jargon capable of confusing the sense should be avoided. Therefore, in the plain language of common sense I now address my readers, and had I the ability to do otherwise, I think I should be inclined to overcome the temptation of using a more attractive style, for fear I should become obscure, and lose the chance of being useful.

Scarcely any two bodies are formed alike, or any two minds alike constituted; every human frame is distinguished by some peculiarity, and many circumstances may occur through life to change our temperament from what it originally was. Most persons must be aware, that a sudden change from affluence to adversity, and "other ills which flesh is heir to," will change the whole mass of blood; the stomach (always sympathizing with every other organ of the body) becomes disordered, the appetite bad, and bowels irregular; every meal is at tended by acidity and a flatulent distension of the stomach; the spirits are depressed; the sufferer becomes irritable, and those feelings influence the healthy qualities of the blood. Then, as a matter of course, the nerves, the liver, the spleen, and all other organs of the body, become more or less affected. From such causes, the effects upon the mind are sometimes so distressing, the spirits are so subdued, that the sufferer becomes unfit for the active duties of life. So thought Shakspeare when he said -

> "Infirmity of mind
> Doth make me neglect my office;
> We are not ourselves when nature, being oppressed,

Commands the mind to suffer with the body ”

I much fear — nay, I have reason to know—that such distressing feelings have caused many persons who otherwise might have continued useful members of society, to attempt their own life, or actually to destroy themselves. We had, in 1836, a case to prove this, *viz.* Mr. Stannynought, of the Edgeware Road, who in a fit of despondency from the causes I have here mentioned, (for I have made diligent enquiry into the case,) destroyed his darling son, and attempted his own life, which on a second attempt he accomplished. Read how beautifully Shakspeare describes a man in such a state -

“Some strange commotion
Is in his brain- he bites his lip, and starts;
Stops on a sudden, looks on the ground,
Then, lays his finger on his temple - straight
Springs out into fast steps — then stops again;
Strikes his breast hard - and then he casts
His eye against the moon; in most strange postures
We have seen him set himself.”

Read the pompous life of Cardinal Wolsey in Shakspeare's Henry the Eighth; he says -

“My high-blown pride
At length broke under me, and now has left me
Weary, and old with service, to the mercy
Of a rude stream."

And what did this rude stream? why caused his stomach to act so powerfully with his distress of mind, that every reflecting person who reads his life, must come, I think, to the conclusion that I have, *viz.* that he died from indigestion, commonly supposed to be, and called a broken heart. The words he made use of would be the effect of an irritable, anxious, and desponding state of mind, caused by his Royal Master giving him a paper in an angry mood, and saying -

“Read o'er this — and after, this - and
Then to breakfast with what appetite you may.”

This act caused him to exclaim

“Had I but served my God with half the zeal
I served my king, he would not in my age
Have left me naked to my enemies.”

"Father Abbot,
An old man broken with the storms of state,
is come to lay his weary bones among you,
Give him a little earth for charity.”
                              SHAKSPEARE.

But such an irritable, anxious, and desponding state of mind as Wolsey's is not always attributable to indigestion; but too often the effects brought on from such a cause as late, formal, and ill-assorted dinners, the extremes of which cause the stomach to ferment instead of digest; for

"Boundless intemperance
In nature is a tyranny; it hath been
The untimely emptying of the happy throne,
And fall of many kings."

"Unquiet meals make ill digestion."
SHAKSPEARE.

This may be perceived by frequent belchings after dinner. This gas does not arise from digestion but fermentation, and may be fitly compared to the fumes which arise from a tub of beer when at work, and it is only necessary to inspect the curd in the stomach of a kitten, to prove that the gastric fluid is an acid. But it differs from the acids human chemistry afford, which are caustic, and destroy the texture of the living body. This difference is indeed wonderful, and, like every other provision of the Deity, is a subject worthy of our consideration and admiration. This gastric fluid, or, more properly to name it, this inimitable liquor, is also a solvent, which acts upon all matters proper for nutrition; and the vitality of the stomach alone secures it from its corrosive power.

Again the Bile, —this is a thick, viscid, soapy fluid, of a yellow colour, and very bitter; it acts no doubt upon the matter of the diluted chyle, and by its peculiar stimulus compels the bowels to urge it onward to the large intestine. The connexion this has with the gall bladder is another work of serious consideration, to inquire for the occasion that demands its use. This remark I am led to make by Shakspeare making Hamlet say:

"Sure I am pigeoned, livered, and lack gall,
To make oppression bitter."

Yet it is worthy of remark, that animals, &c. who do not fast long, -as the horse,—the parrot, -- and the pigeon - have not any gall bladder; this must account for the food passing so soon through the body, as it could not long remain without being in an acrid and fermenting state, from want of the bitter mixed with the fluids in the bowels, which no doubt the gall bladder supplies. Again the barrel of ale affords us a proof that bitters resist fermentation and putrefaction, for without the bitter of the hop, the infusion of malt would soon become vinegar. In the same manner the bile, seasoned with the bitter from the gall bladder, prevents the corruption of the contents of nature's passage from the stomach onwards. These things working so truly together, and being ordained with so much apparent foresight, can we for one moment doubt whether they are the effects of *chance* (as an able writer will have it), or the Providence of a Merciful God, who in mercy afflicts us with disease, to convince us we must obey the general laws of nature established by himself? In attempting to explain these things, I consider myself as composing a solemn hymn to the Author of our Bodily Frame: I first strive, by a persevering inquiry and study, to comprehend these things myself, and next I endeavour to show them to others, to evidence to them how great is the Deity's wisdom, goodness, and mercy. Deducing my own opinion from these reflections, I have traced many of the cases brought under my notice, (particularly patients in the higher ranks of life,) to the inconsiderate sacrifices made to fashion and custom, at the laborious dinner table! Luxurious and extravagant dinners produce suffering rather than enjoyment, as they are contrary to the laws of human nature. Let us for a moment take a view of the (to say the least of it) insane fashion of drinking *healths* in *wine* at the dinner table. I have always contended that the thing was so absurd that it must have been brought into fashion by a drunkard. On enquiry, I found I was right, and, poor man, his sufferings before his death made him pay dear for this folly.

A very old author (Malbranch) tells us, that our senses were given us to guard ourselves from injuries, and that they never fail to answer the end for which they were given. If this good old man could but come amongst us again, and see one of our fashionable dinners, he would at once be startled at our lack of common sense, which tells us, that when extremes such as they generally consist of meet in the human stomach, a sort of Bubble-and-squeak contest takes place, Mr. Acid endeavouring with all his might to turn Mr. Saccharine-juice out of the house by forcing him up the chimney; -if he fails in this, he disturbs his healthy body with a diseased fluid, or fills the system with vinegar and grease. This was the case with Royalty itself. Had *he* paid attention to the remarks of that eminent man Dr. Hunter, he would have found that: - "The stomach gives information when the supplies have been expended, and represents with great exactness the quantity and quality of whatever is wanted in the present state of the machine, and in proportion as it meets with neglect or disappointment, rises or falls in its demand."

> "He that in health would long remain,
> From drinking healths he must refrain"

The spirit of the said wine mixing with the juices of the stomach and food, forms a fluid that prevents the absorbents from taking up and conveying the nutriment to the body; likewise the spirit acting upon the nerves, causes them to lose their elasticity. We know the bow, over-bent, becomes good for nothing; and the nerves being of an elastic nature, when over-pressed and excited by large quantities of wine, at last lose their tone, and instead of extending become relaxed, lose their wonted vigour, and are not able to disburden themselves of the morbid particles cast upon them. This brings to mind an opinion I once heard expressed by a very clever lecturer; it so pleased me that I took his words down. He said, "should the Body sue the Mind before a court of judicature for damages, it would be found that the Mind would prove a ruinous tenant to its landlord. " And how can this be otherwise, as in these days man is ignorant of himself! All his boasted education has not taught him the constituent elements of his own nature; he, of course, acts entirely at random, and exposes himself to innumerable miseries, —which, by knowing the component parts of himself, might have been avoided. By knowing that the "proper study of mankind is man," he will not fail quickly to perceive, that on considering the construction of his body, and the necessity of healthy fluids to maintain health, he will at once see the danger of intemperance, both in eating and drinking — for if the vital functions are not regularly performed by a proper state of the solids and fluids, our health must be impaired, digestion hurt, -nerves relaxed, -secretions irregular, -and, as a natural consequence, disease must ensue. From experience I can state that but few, comparatively speaking, regard this, though claiming the title of reasonable, rational beings; yet with professions on their tongue, they become slaves to their appetites by perpetually searching out something to gratify their artificial wants.

"Take heed lest your hearts be overcharged with surfeiting and drunkeness." - Luke xxi. 34.

By eating, Adam lost Paradise, and Esau his birth-right. I beg my readers to remember the wise maxim , that - "we do not live to eat and drink, but eat and drink to live." Eat, then, only to support nature, to preserve health, and to prolong life, not to destroy it. As to drink, I would recommend the advice of St. Paul, "Brethren be sober and watchful:" if not we lay ourselves open to attacks of our enemies, for there are plenty of Iago's in this world who might say with him:

> "If I can fasten but one cup upon him,
> With that which he hath drunk to -night already,
> He'll be as full of quarrel and offence,
> As my young mistress's lap-dog:"

And when, like Cassio, we have fallen into the trap of our foes, we may with him when too late exclaim,

"I remember a mass of things
But nothing distinctly — a quarrel—
But nothing wherefore- O that
Men should put an enemy in their
Mouths, to steal away their brains!
I will ask him for my place,
He shall tell me-I am a drunkard;
Had I as many mouths as Hydra,
Such an answer would stop them all;
To be now a sensible man, by and bye a fool,
And presently a beast! O strange,
Every inordinate cup is unblessed,
And the ingredient is a devil."

Nature is content with little, but luxury knows no bounds; and Aristotle tells us that common sense is a blessing and a virtue, for it is necessary to the young mind, comfortable to the aged, serviceable to the poor, an ornament to the rich, an honour to the fortunate, and a support to the unfortunate. Yet common sense points out to us that Nature delights in plain and simple food, and every animal, except man, obeys her dictates. But man, the lord of the world, the head of the visible creation, has the wretched prerogative of transgressing the laws prescribed to his exalted nature by the wisest hand! Is not this a blind impulse? This would not be the case if the education of youth were built on the knowledge of God and his works. The practice of these studies would vegetate, and show the foundation on which all just judgment of mankind should be built. Strange! that the sufferings and sudden deaths which are daily occasioned by intemperance, should have so little effect on the lovers of the bottle and the banquet! I believe that nearly every malady is brought on, by high-ways or bye-ways, from an over-loaded stomach; and when I have seen a fashionable practitioner mysteriously counting the pulse of his patient, or with a silver spoon on the tongue looking down his red and inflamed gullet, I have felt disposed to exclaim, "why not feel his skin, it is a much better monitor than the pulse? " tell your patient, "Sir, you have lived improperly; you have eaten too much, drank too much, and sat too much. Look, Sir, at the savages, who live actively and temperately-- they have only one great disorder - death; this is a sufficient proof that the human frame was not created imperfect; it is we ourselves that have made it so." I know I shall be blamed for bringing before the mind of wealthy people any truth which may be unpalatable to them; many would rather go on stuffing their beds with the thorns of pain and bitter reflection, instead of the down of repose and comfort, and when lying on the former, they writhe and groan with the agony they have inflicted on themselves. Now, to guard against this it is necessary for us to consider, as near as our senses and reasonable deductions will carry us, the nature of the threads and fibres of which the solids of a human body are composed. Engaged in this contemplation, I have often observed with admiration the wisdom and goodness of Providence, in furnishing such wonderful antidotes in our happy land for all the diseases of an English constitution and climate, where diseases are chiefly owing to errors of diet, or rather, as a sacred writer expresses it, - "to idleness, and fulness of bread;" the living so much on meat - the inconstancy of the weather, our sedentary amusements; yet, to remedy all which, kind Heaven has provided sovereign restoratives and preventatives for all our ills, and it is the duty of man to study their use and properly apply them. Patients are very apt to inquire of their medical attendants, "What is my disease? " A true answer to this question is not always convenient, nor would it be pleasing to the inquirer, therefore he gratifies his patient with a general term: "Madam or Sir, you are bilious." This is very satisfactory, and often pleasing to persons of fashion, as they claim an exclusive privilege to this supposed disease, brought into note by a fashionable apothecary, who had often been puzzled for an answer to the inquiries of his patients. Had I not witnessed the mischief this fashionable term has caused, by increasing consumption and scrofula, I should not have attempted (as I intend) to be at some pains to point out the danger of taking medicine to carry off this supposed offensive bile; this bad habit tends to destroy the health they wish to preserve. In giving my reasons for believing that illness in ninety cases out of every hundred proceeds from the deficiency of bile, it will be proper to consider the meaning of the term bilious. I have no doubt that the bile discharged is more frequently the effect, than the cause of redundancy, brought on from the want of sleep and rest at the seasons intended by the God of Nature; also from the want of exercise, and the uncongenial food and drink we take. Persons of relaxed, delicate, or dissipated habits, generally complain of excess of bile, when the very reverse is the case - for this reason; the weakness of their vital powers occasions a languor of the circulation - consequently this produces a poor and a watery state of the blood; the secreted humours, the bile particularly, is much less pungent than it ought to be. Other causes will produce the same effect. The suffering poor, who are reduced by indigence, improper diet, or disease, often labour under the same defect of the bile, and this continues until they are better fed, when they recover a sufficiency of bile in proportion as they gain strength. Here is one of the beautiful provisions of nature, that she is always ready to supply or take away, as may be necessary, and provides for the restoration of health, if she be kindly treated. In fever, I have no doubt, the gall bladder, from the heat of the body, becomes inactive, or else why do we so soon lose our appetites and the sensitive palate? The reason I think is plain; it is well understood that there are thousands of absorbing vessels always employed in taking up and conveying the juices for the nutriment of the body, in time of fever in all its kinds; those vessels are wanted for another use, namely, to act the very reverse to their employment in health; instead of taking up, they are wanted as drains, to convey the diseased fluid into the different channels, to be expelled from the body. But there are many diseases accompanied with a sallow complexion, or what is called a bilious tinge of the skin. It is for the want of this necessary ingredient (as many of the articles of our food are of a tough, glutinous and viscid nature) that the digestive power of the stomach cannot completely assimilate its contents; the bile contributes, by its soapy quality, very much to complete the necessary change, and at the same time excites the absorbing vessels or lacteals to carry it into circulation. Even in diseases of the liver (the organ which prepares the bile), it does not, strictly speaking, deserve the name of bilious. A bitter taste of the mouth, a brownish fur on the tongue, a sickness and sense of oppression at the pit of the stomach, are believed to be undoubted proofs of offensive bile in the stomach, especially if it be discharged by vomiting. Yet this is not surprising when we consider the unnatural mixture of food which is swallowed in a day. Here lies the grand fault, not in the wholesome bile, for had that continued in the stomach, its assimilating quality would rather have prevented those unnatural ferments, than have caused them. And no doubt this was the office nature intended it to perform, for after the food is passed onwards into the bowels, if the some fermentable action was to take place in the small intestines which occurs in the stomach (which the bile prevents), they would burst, and society could not long exist, under the present system of diet.

Most persons believe that bile is necessary to the stomach, to assist the digestion of our food; I would ask those who entertain such a supposition, by what chance did it get there? for if the bile ever gets into the stomach, it must be by a perverted and opposite motion of the bowels, and contrary to gravity - which, being contrary to the simplicity of the operations of nature, cannot easily be admitted, for if the wise Author of our Being had intended that the bile should be part of the digestive fluid of the stomach, it might as easily have been conveyed there by a small tube or pipe, similar to the ureters which convey the water from the kidneys to the bladder. Some may ask (and with some plausability), how can bile be discharged from the stomach if it never gets there? The answer is easy, and as easily understood; the great sensation of sickness from a foul stomach causes a regurgitation of bile into the stomach, by inverting and counteracting the natural motion of the bowels or intestine which is closely connected with the stomach. Hence it often happens that, from its very soapy quality, pure bile is discharged by the first effort, and so always increases in quantity as the stomach gets empty; this is no proof of its being the offending cause of the vomiting, but an accidental effect. I was at sea off Torbay a few years since, with about 250 persons on a pleasure excursion by steam, and, with the exception of my brother (whom I had prepared for the voyage) and myself, there was scarcely one who was not dreadfully sick. Read Shakspeare's description of that painful sensation:

"But still the envious flood
Kept in my soul, and would not let it forth,
But smothered it within my panting body,
Which almost burst to belch it in the sea.

SHAKSPEARE.

Some of the party I had known from "my boyish days, " and never knew them to have had any illness; and as I like to take advantage of every circumstance that will employ and improve my mind, I particularly watched those persons, and found they threw up a larger quantity of bile than any three of the unhealthy ones, whose constitutions I likewise knew. It was this incident that first drew my attention to the subject, for on our landing, they came in a body to return me thanks for the kindness I had considered it my duty to pay them, by holding up their heads and drenching them with warm water, to expedite their cure. I embraced this opportunity to inquire into the state of health and constitution of many that I had not previously known, and found that those who suffered most, and threw up least bile, had been told by their doctors (and firmly believed it themselves), that they were bilious, and were continually taking blue pills and black draughts, to remove that from the body they were actually in want of. These pernicious medicines not only carry away the healthy bile, but also the digestive mucus or lining of the stomach, which kind nature has placed there, to *rot* (that is the English word) the food we eat; the consequence is, that when these rich juices of many sorts, mixed together beyond the conception of man, are carried off, the stomach, by sympathy for the want of it, collapses or contracts; the palate of the mouth, which is part of the stomach, sympathizes with its friend, and loses its relish for food; and should art be used to tempt the stomach to receive any, there it lays like a lump of lead, causing spasms, heart-burn, head-ache, &c. &c. &c. for several days, as it cannot digest for the want of nature's cordial. During this time there is no action of the bowels - the tongue becomes furred, the skin dry, and while the poor sufferer is wishing for death, the doctor is called in, and his blue pill remedy is again applied, which had before been the cause of all the mischief. A repetition of this sort, in my opinion, is the cause of man's degenerating in personal strength at about the same rate as he is increasing in general intellect; and I cannot assign any other cause for the great increase of scrofula, dropsy, and consumption, which an observing mind must have noticed have for many years been making sad inroads upon the constitution of the British people. I was about to prove that the colour of the skin, or even throwing up bile, is no proof that a person is bilious. In Devonshire, when a boy, I have witnessed, in the old practice of wrestling, that from the dreadful kicks a fine healthy young man has received, he has thrown up abundance of bile. A blow on the head, or a sudden fright, will produce the same effect; and that bile never passes into the stomach unless the action of vomiting brings it there, which gives a stronger shake to the whole system (solid and fluid,) than any other motion will be found capable of. Let any of my readers observe, and they will find the last products of vomiting will discover a drain of humours, brought into the stomach from some considerable distance in the bowels, and the colour of some part of it will show it comes from the liver, as, on dissection, such will be found in those parts. Vomiting is one of nature's own contrivances to throw- up what is offensive to the stomach, which is often so extremely sour as even to corrode the throat. Now if bile had been constantly present in the stomach it would have neutralised and corrected this sharp acid, which may be proved by mixing ox gall with any acid. The idea of bile being a prominent cause of disease is a gross and foolish error, and in its consequences, as every day proves, a very injurious one; and the attempt to carry off this most useful and salutary humour, when it is already too scanty, is likely to lead, and frequently does lead, to most dangerous and fatal consequences. Had Abernethy lived a hundred years, and done good the whole time, he never could have atoned for the injury done to his fellow creatures by teaching them to take blue pill. Read his book, and there it will be found recommended as a cure for every disease. I have yet to learn if this was not *Quackery* in its *true* meaning. It is wonderful that a man of so much learning should recommend so gross an absurdity, that one remedy on all constitutions (where no two are alike), should be capable of restoring the tone of the fibres when they are too weak, and relax them when too rigid; that it should give substance to the fluids when too watery, and liquify them when they are too viscid; that it should calm the nerves when in a state of excitement, and restore to them their proper tone when they are inert. Such a practice surely can only require a moment's reflection, to perceive its absurdity; it is the abuse, and not the use of mercury that I condemn, for I have no doubt, in some constitutious and disorders, it may be used with the bath with great success, but during its operation the patient ought not to leave the bed-room. Thousands are now living who fancy they cannot be well unless under the specific action of mercury, which must prove injurious, as it keeps them susceptible to colds — which more or less are the fore runners to all our ailments:-Shakspeare says

"The evil that men do - lives after them. "

So it is with Abernethy, and those who walk in his steps. They never can reflect on the truth of the homely proverb, "what is one man's meat, is another's poison." My opinion is the same of both medicine and diet; both must be adapted to the exigencies of nature, and all other circumstances which an attentive eye and mind will always observe. It would be as absurd for all men to diet alike, or to take the same medicines, *even for the same disease*, as it would be for all men to wear the same sized clothes, hats, or shoes. To the worshippers of this practice I have in this work given a friendly recipe. Such as will not try it, I would recommend to attend to Lord Byron's, who prescribes for all opium and Pil. Hydrag. takers, — " go read your bible, pray, and mind your purse."

Persons who are troubled with indigestion, -or who have weak stomachs, ought to live by rule, avoiding pastry, unripe fruits, pickles, and every thing that is flatulent, or in its nature fermentable and hard of digestion. They should pay a more than ordinary attention to their mode of diet : they should eat little and often, and then only from one dish at a meal, such as boiled mutton or fowl, with the decoction commonly called broth, particularly the produce of over-boiled animal food, which contains all the richness of the meat. It may be said this remedy has often been tried and found unavailing: but it is not its adoption for a day, week, or month, that will improve the patient, or remove the cause it must be done imperceptibly; nature must not be hurried - she must have her own time to re establish her own fluids in her digestive cistern, (for so we might call the stomach). I should say not less than six, and in very desperate cases, twelve months, this ought to be fairly tried, and those who, from long suffering, can value and appreciate the blessing of health and comfort, (for without this all other temporal blessings are as lost,) must, or at least ought to submit to this system, as the only means capable of accomplishing the removal of those troublesome diseases, brought on by improper medical treatment or the habits of diet of the present *era* - or most likely by a little of both.

Another great evil is, that persons finding themselves improve by this rule of regimen and diet, by their own suggestion or that of their friends, they indulge in some very foolish and extravagant luxury; the consequence is, they knock down all they have built up, like a new wall receiving a shock before the mortar is set: this for a time brings them to exercise their common sense, and they go on regularly until they again feel their improvement, when they have another treat, as it is called, which brings on another attack; this often repeated tries their patience, till at last, they give up in despair, and leave the cause of the complaint to triumph, and this only for the want of perseverance and firmness. Then the poor stomach is blamed because it does not do double and treble the duty that nature intended it should, and they would rather continue with all their sufferings, than be deprived of what they falsely call the comforts of life. To such I trust I am not now devoting my time; I must leave them to "those thorns that in their bosoms lodge," to shrink and struggle under the effects of their own folly. But this shall not prevent me from probing the cause from the foundation, for I now feel myself in that responsible situation in life, that lays upon me a great obligation, not only to make known the curative art, but also that which is by far the best, *viz.* the preventative: which I intend to do for the benefit of the afflicted.

Every person ought to be as conversant with their own constitution as they are with the language of their country; then they would know from experience what food, drink, and mode of living is the most agreeable to their constitution, and as these change at different periods of life, they would find that what agrees with them at one time, will disagree at another. This is not surprising when we consider how many reasons may be assigned, as age, weather - easy or unhappy state of the mind - if this should be worried or troubled more than the body, the latter trembles and languishes, becomes disturbed, and sinks beneath itself.

Many, by excessive application, to study, render their bodies sickly and unfit to bear its own burden. *Celsus* tells us that "men ought to eat a great deal of meat", but he adds this caution, "provided they can digest it;" - which cannot be expected by those who call off the natural heat of the stomach every hour to assist the offices of the mind. This I myself often feel, and when I am quite exhausted and worn out with fatigue, and would give the world for one hour's rest, I comfort myself as if I already possessed the ease and quiet I so much longed for. I have just sufficient wisdom to know that I must not neglect the body for the exclusive improvement of the mind; to make both work well, they must be kept on an even balance; like landlord and tenant, they must each act for their mutual advantage, and not trample each other under foot; and although the mind has but one disease, yet that disease is equal to all the body's afflictions. This my favourite author has shewn; such as: - "The griping pains, ruptures, catarrhs, loads of the gravel in the back, lethargies, palsies, raw eyes, rotten livers, wheezing lungs, bladders full of imposthume, sciaticus, lime-kilns in the palm, incurable bone ache, rivetted fee simple of the tetter,

"Joints of every thing,
But every thing so out of
Joint - that he is a gouty Briareus,
Many hands of no use."

I think few men have suffered more from an over anxious working of the mind than I have. I remember that, but a few years since, I could digest any thing in the shape of good nourishing food, drink beer, wine, or spirits, and eat hot meat suppers, without feeling any ill effects. - But for the last seven years, although in the prime of life, my close and intense study, and diligent application to the patients under my care, (for when my limbs are resting themselves on the bed or couch, the head is working in contriving the best means for tomorrow, and as I know man is as incapable of continual thought, as he is of continual exercise, I find, by drawing too much on the bank of knowledge,) has so much impaired my digestive powers, that I am now compelled to live on very light food, yet of a nourishing nature. If I was to take one glass of ale with my dinner, it would for hours make me quite miserable. There is no general rule to be laid down for these effects, and no individual must stand up for them on a universal principle. Exceptions must always be made, to adopt that course which the patient's constitution requires; by such means much mischief in the digestive process" might be prevented without any medicine, simply by knowing the cause.

But system of diet alone, however well adjusted, both in quantity and quality, will not answer the end, without moderate bodily exercise, for our bodies are so made, and the animal economy so contrived that, without exercise, the juices will thicken, the joints stiffen, the nerves relax, and the digestive powers become weakened. The natural constitution of man is wonderful indeed, to endure the changes and irregularities that we impose upon it; this blessing and advantage arises from the wonderful communications of internal parts which act by that necessity of sympathy, that when one part is affected, another comes immediately to its relief. Yet for all this a change of diet may be very useful, according to circumstances and the seasons. Nature teaches us this by the vast variety of food which she has provided for man, and it is his duty to study a good adjustment thereof for the digestive powers, and such as will well keep pace with what is expended in motion, excrement, effluvia, ***** (sic), for if any man gratifies his taste beyond the limits of prudence, he knows not where it may end.

He that begins with a sparrow, may end with a hawk. - If concoction or digestion be impaired by our folly, we must beware of adding more heavy food upon such crudities, for when crude juices are mixed one with the other, we may think ourselves fortunate if we can discharge them by the ordinary evacuations; in such a case, even one meal a day would be too much if chosen of improper meats. We ought to take (with proper medicine, such as I shall here recommend) pure and light food, and such as is familiar to the constitution and disposition: for it is the same with food, as with other likes and dislikes, some are more acceptable than others, to act in unison with the mind, the stomach, and the palate. It would be waste of time for me to write (or others read), to recommend one particular food for all indiscriminately, for sometimes one description of food compared with that of another, although in some respects inferior, is overbalanced by the inclination of the appetite towards it. And this ought not to seem strange but very reasonable, when we consider how we all differ in personal appearance, disposition, and constitution, from each other. Shakspeare, in his masterly way, has shewn us that this is another wise provision of nature, in his "Comedy of Errors." What confusion and miserable wretchedness we should all be in, if any two of us were born alike! I have often thought, if it was only this one act of God's providence, it is enough to satisfy any unbeliever that there exists a Supreme Being, who saw the evils that would arise, from such a similarity. My readers will see I am often drawn into such like observations when shewing the different effects which food, disease, and medicine, have on each of us. As I take nature for my guide, I cannot go on without her assistance.

> "Untune this string and see what discord follows!
> Tyranny plucks justice by the nose,
> The baby beats the nurse,
> And quite athwart goes all decorum."
> > - SHAKSPEARE.

See the universal sympathy of the stomach with every part of the living body, particularly that of the skin. There is a peculiar dry and contracted state of the skin - this is always a sure indication of a deranged state of the digestive organs, and a state which I have always found gradually disappear under some mild and natural treatment, with out the use of mercury. The clearness of the complexion is the best proof of a man's being in good condition. I wish the profession studied this art more, or even as well as those who understand and direct the system of training or treatment of horses.

I shall now give the results of my practice upon the subject of Indigestion. I am encouraged in this duty by a conviction of the advantage which will arise to the sufferer from acting on the system I am about to recommend, over that of the destructive mercurial practice.

> "Be comforted -
> Let's make us medicine of our great revenge
> To cure this deadly grief."
> > SHAKSPEARE.

And I promise that, on a fair trial, it will be found that the means I have recommended will be all that is necessary to cleanse a foul stomach, and strengthen it, without any deleterious effects. No thing will give me greater pleasure than to find that my readers have derived benefit from this advice, as I give it without any other fee than that indescribable pleasure every man feels in the act of doing good.

> " I gave it freely ever — and there is none
> Can truly say he gives, if he receiveṣ.
> If our betters play at that game - we must not dare
> To imitate them.
> Ceremony was but devised at first

To set a gloss on faint deeds.   Hollow welcome -
Recanting goodness
But where there is true friendship - there needs none."

 Then here I give no other advice than that which tends to the good of mankind - well knowing if it be faithfully and skilfully used, it will be found capable of performing much more than ever I have promised. I am borne out in this opinion, by the success attending my own practice, and also by the concurrent testimony of multitudes of medical and scientific men from all parts of England.

Shakspeare, in describing the life of a man, has divided it into seven stages of ten years each. I think, with such a medical mind as he had, he might have subdivided the seven into about fifteen, as I have no doubt in every stage hereafter mentioned, a change or alteration in the bodily frame takes place; and this agrees with what I have said on the action of medicine on different constitutions and periods of life. When a child is seven days old it is disencumbered of the remains of the navel-string; at twice seven days it notices the light; at thrice seven days observes objects, and follows them with its eyes; at seven months the teeth begin to appear; at twice seven months usually it begins to walk; at thrice seven months begins to utter words; at four times seven months walks alone; at seven years, the teeth are renewed; at twice seven years the beard begins to grow; at three times seven years the body attains full growth; at four times seven life is in perfection; and until five times seven remains so; at six times seven the strength and health begin to fail; at seven times seven the mind attains maturity; ten times seven is the full age of man; after which (there are a few happy exceptions) he is then only fit for the crutches made by Dame Nature for declining life, which are quietness and retirement. This gives him an opportunity of looking back on an idle and wicked, or a well - spent life, and to feel that although he has lived in a crowd, he must soon die by himself. He reasons thus: - "I have proved that youth is not the age of pleasure; we then expect too much, and are therefore daily exposed to disappointments and mortifications — for this reason, that seldom any thing happens in this life precisely to our wishes, and properly so too. When we get a little older, and have brought down our wishes to our experience, then we become calm and begin to enjoy ourselves: but this feeling can only be felt by the good and happy. It is hardly necessary for me to state, that the doses I have prescribed must very frequently be varied in quantity, according to the effects they produce; it is time and observation only, that can teach invalids those essential things. I would advise, as my own system of treatment, to begin with small doses, and increase them as the constitution will bear, and remember that it is better to have ten failures from over cautiousness, than to risk the loss of one life from rashness. The means I here recommend are such as are easily obtained, and safe even in unskilful hands. Many herbs that I use being scarce, I grow them myself. As regards others not named, it would be unsafe to recommend their indiscriminate use.

I shall first commence with a remedy for a diseased stomach, such as is commonly described as bilious, and for which the blue pill is said to be the sovereign remedy. It will be seen that my great aim is to reduce medicine to so simple a form that every individual may attend to his general health himself, without having recourse to the delusions of quackery, or the equally absurd practice of mysterious pretenders to college medical science. The patient ought to feel and know that when any part of the body becomes painful, or when he feels sick and giddy, or low - spirited without a cause, and loses all appetite for food, I say he ought to know that there is something wrong in the system. Let him first attend to the stomach and take,

No. 1

One ounce of Mountain Flax,
One ditto of Senna Leaves,
Four ditto of Liquorice Root,
One do. Rosemary (if agreeable to palate);

boil these in two quarts of water for two hours, strain when cold, and drink a wine-glass full morning, noon, and night. This combination is such a searcher to the system that it seldom acts on the bowels under twelve or sixteen hours; during that time it causes a little sickness, or nausea in the stomach; let this be continued for a week, unless the bowels become too active, then rest for a day or two, and go on again. By these means the liver will be purged and cleansed, and at the same time prevent the accumulation of fæculent matter in the colon. On the second week, if all goes on well (say three or four active and easy motions on a strong person, or half that number on a debilitated one), I would recommend

No. 2.

One ounce of dried Marsh Mallow,
Half ditto of Mountain Flax,
One ditto of Carduous or Holy Thistle,
One ditto of the herb Chirayita;

boil these in a quart of water for one hour, strain it into a jug, and when reduced to about sixty degrees, next add to it two drachms of dried carbonate of soda.   Dose: a wine-glass full noon and night for about another week; this will strengthen the stomach, produce healthy chyle, stimulate the whole mass of blood, and keep the bowels in a regular state.   On the third week I should recommend infusions instead of decoctions, for I consider that in the latter preparation many of the fine particles and essential oils pass off by evaporation. The herbs hereafter named ought to be taken about three times a week, until the system is re-established by the enjoyment of health. Should occasion require, as it will do in long-standing cases, he must return back to prescription No. 1 and 2, as before.

Infusion for giving a tone to the stomach. Take
No. 3 .

Four drachms of best Rhubarb Root, bruised,
Four ditto of dried Ground Ivy, bruised,
Two ditto of Gentian Root, bruised,
Two ditto of Ginger Root, bruised,
Two ditto of fresh Lemon Peel;

pour on these one quart of boiling water in a clean well-covered earthen jug, let it stand twenty -four hours, strain first through a coarse cloth or sieve, then through clean muslin, and take a wine glass full at noon and night. Not more than a pint or quart should be made for one person at a time, and then both this and the decoction should be kept well corked. I always use distilled water for decoctions and infusions, but to those who cannot get it, clean rain water, or pure river water, boiled several hours before used, is best for extracting the virtue from all kinds of herbs. Spring water should never be used. If these simple directions are attended to, any of my readers may make it in every respect as well as the first chemist in England. The best vessel for boiling ingredients for decoctions in, is about a three-pint or two- quart tin tea kettle, which should be kept for this purpose; anything of copper should be avoided. If the patient is very low, I would advise

No. 4.

One ounce of dried Mint,
Two drachms of Rhubarb Root,
One ditto of Cinnamon;

pour on them one pint of water; after twenty-four hours, strain. This quantity may be taken in two days. Should it not agree well on the stomach, take,

No.5.

Gentian Root, half an ounce,
Peruvian Bark, ditto,
Orange Peel, two drachms,
White Cinnamon, one ditto;

let these be infused in one bottle of good sherry wine, and take a wine-glass full every day at noon. This may not agree with many who for a long time have been suffering from a dry cough; to such I would advise

Two ounces of Linseed,
Four ditto of Liquorice Root,
Four ditto of Sun Raisins,
Two quarts of soft water;

let these simmer over a slow fire until reduced to one quart, then strain, and add to it half a pound of honey. Take half a pint in three doses every day, with about a dessert-spoonful of rum or brandy to each dose.

Or take the following, which is an excellent warm medicine for the aged. Take of the best senna, one ounce, jalap, coriander (or carroway seeds) bruised, and cream of tartar, each half an ounce, sugar candy powdered six ounces, dried sub-carbonate of soda one drachm, old rum or brandy, one pint and a half; let it stand in a warm place for a fortnight; often shaking it, strain off, and take a dessert-spoonful twice a day.

This is an excellent remedy for a weak constitution; very pleasant for a gentle purge, and is so easily made that it may always be kept for family use. Many may not be enabled to get the strengthening herbs; to such , I would recommend the following tincture to strengthen the organs of digestion:

Tincture of Virginia Snake Root,
Ditto of Columbia Root,
Compound ditto of Cardamom Seeds,
Compound Tincture of Bark,

of each one ounce; mix and take two or three tea-spoonsful every day, one hour before and after dinner, in a wine-glass full of mint tea. Drink speedwell and wood betony for breakfast and tea, instead of foreign tea. All that I have here recommended will be unavailing unless the feet are kept clean and warm, with plenty of room in the shoe for the blood to circulate. If this be not attended to, the feet become cold, and have neither spring or play in their movement.

Many persons have applied to me with corns, bunions, and weak ankles, and I have at once seen that by wearing their shoes *rights and lefts,* and much too small, that the whole weight of their bodies have been borne by just the outside of the heel and one side of the foot, thereby throwing the sustaining bone of the ankle out of its natural perpendicular, and causing it to lose its focus and equilibrium. A slender stick whilst upright will support a great weight, which when bent will sink under it; it is the same with the ankle when erect - it is able to bear the weight of the body; this, in either sex, has the most injurious effects on the supporting ankles. To such I always recommend strait shoes, and the changing them every day, for I have always found it to be a cure for weak ankles, and often assists me in the cure of bodily disease. Follow the multitude in the streets, see how they tread, and then place an infant on the table, and observe the difference of the position of the foot and ankle; the latter is nature — the former pride and folly.

The same remarks apply to the fair sex, on the evils of tight- lacing, an evil which brings on palpitation of the heart, short breathing, head-aches, consumption, and funerals without number; these are the daily results of following the milliners' contracted patterns. Who would wish the heart, the lungs, the liver, the kidneys, the bowels (the length of which are six times that of the body) which it is very well known frequently to contain eight pounds of solid mass — all these and much more to be barrelled and squeezed up in little more than the circumference of a quart pot! Such a narrow waist is often too dearly purchased by loss of health and deformity of person, and all this for the purpose of being, as it is so foolishly called, genteel, against the laws of nature!   Let sickness and disease once predominate over the beauteous form of woman, and the snowy whiteness of the skin is exchanged for a sallow hue, the brightness of the eyes tarnished, and the blooming cheek soon fades.

This pernicious habit will prevent the growth and proper position of the ribs, the muscles, the chest, and the spine, which must all act in harmony, as they are so essential to the required strength of the vertebral column, and the proper freedom of the thoracic and digestive organs; and I can assure my fair young friends, that the caution I have here given must not be trifled or tampered with; I have known many fall a sacrifice to its neglect, which makes it the more my duty to raise the warning voice ere it be too late. The thoughtless may say,

“This is the very coinage of your brain,
This bodiless creation Ecstasy
Is very cunning in,”

To such I would answer:

“My pulse, as yours, doth temperately keep time,
And makes as healthful music. It is not madness
That I have uttered: bring me to the test,
And I the matter will explain - which madness
Cannot do.
Lay not that flattering unction to your soul,
It will but skin and film the ulcerous place;
Whiles rank corruption, festering all within,
Infects unseen.
Repent what's past; avoid what is to come;
And do not spread, the compost on the weeds,
To make them ranker. "
                    SHAKSPEARE.

Had I merely discovered the virtues of the Holy Thistle which I have communicated to the public, in my last edition, with the greatest plainness and sincerity, I had certainly even in this "done the state some service". This simple herb is a cure and preventative for those peculiarly distressing feelings arising from the *Vapours, Nervous disorders* of all kinds, hysterical affections brought on by the solids being relaxed and weak, and when a proper regimen of diet and exercise had not been observed - the consequence will be, that digestion will be imperfect. The absorbing vessels of the stomach, instead of running healthy fluids, will become gross and gluey. The glands, and internal coats of the intestines, will become loaded and distended with wind (or, more properly speaking, gas), where by sharp, sour, ill-conditioned fumes, steams, and vapours will be constantly ascending to the brain, to cause head-ache, giddiness, and oppression of spirits to discompose its natural and useful functions, and to paint false and delusive images on the imagination. So that if these effects (their causes I have explained) be allowed to remain, and if proper remedies be not applied, these fumes, wind (or gas), and vapours, get along with the unconcocted and ill- conditioned chyle, through the lacteals, into the blood and other juices; thus the blood becomes thick, and cannot freely circulate.

All the other juices are regulated by the fountain of life - the blood; they become also thick and gluey, and cannot pass by their natural drains through the pores of the skin. This, in my opinion, is the first, on the black list of miseries and sufferings under which so many fellow creatures are now suffering, for the want of that knowledge which ought to be the first rudiments of our education. These causes, and their remedies, being generally known, a knowledge of these important truths would grow with their growth, and prevent men, licensed by Act of Parliament, from making rapid fortunes by trifling with the greatest of all possible blessings - sound Bodily Health. To paraphrase Shakspeare, I would say—

> He that robs me of my health,
> Robs me of that which not enricheth him -
> But makes me poor indeed."

I have often reflected with "sorrow more than anger," when alone, after receiving the visits of men of first -rate ability, well educated, some deeply versed in most arts and sciences, having a general knowledge of life, and reasoning well on the wonderful and perfect works of Nature— yet with all this, they are lamentably deficient in the all important object, namely, that delightful study of themselves, which must in its progress open their eyes, and give them a heart to love and bless God for his wonderful providence in the construction of the human frame; this pleasing study would lay a foundation in the young mind for religious principles, and teach him that he must not only believe the word of God, but also obey it. With their minds thus enlightened — the youth of our noblest families, as well as of our poorest peasantry, might become useful members of society. But, from the faulty system of education followed in England, the former are sent to a public school, the common slaughter-house of the understanding, where they are not "tried and tutored in the world," or in the imbibing knowledge best suited to their youth; but are tied down to the study of nearly useless languages, and the only Geography they learn is, "the world as known to the ancients;" and as a sort of finish they are made to study the rubbish part, by going as it is called "into Ovid," which study will do every thing that human ingenuity could invent, to sully, degrade, and ruin the mind of youth: for there the Almighty Creator of the world is caricatured by a set of gods and goddesses, made grossly licentious! With such instruction, mixt up with the common frailties of our nature, the young mind becomes so puzzled, that it becomes actually unable to distinguish truth from falsehood, or right from wrong; and in this state they are launched into the world as accomplished men, full of the advantages of a good classical education!

Far better would it be to leave the young mind an absolute blank, and rely for morals and profitable instruction in a similar way to those classes whose information and knowledge is enforced on them by the necessities of their daily avocations and necessities. This was the opinion of a worthy man, now living; and perhaps I cannot do better than give his own words, as he wrote from practical experience. He says:-

"Yes, there stands the block, there lies the birch, - that instrument of an immodest and disgraceful punishment; that monument of "ancient night!" Is it not strange that while public opinion is putting an end to corporal punishment in the army, as debasing and brutalising even to the dregs of society, is it not strange, I say, that this punishment should be upheld and applauded as applicable to the feelings and conditions of 'ingenious youth?' As a means of discipline it is notoriously inefficient; no lad of spirit regards for an instant the mere pain of the infliction. It is a point of honour to despise it; and when the sense of its disgrace is overcome, when delicacy is blunted, and shame replaced by effrontery, the influence of the punishment is at an end. But here again the indolence of the master is consulted at the expense of the pupil; it is easier to flog than to teach — it is easier to inflict stripes than to form the character; and accordingly flogging is still the order of the day."

Will flogging, or such a system of education, impress them with any one of the wonderful works of God's providence to man? No, it will misdirect them, and form in them a mind indisposed to study the productions of the earth, and the blessings sent down on them from heaven every moment of their lives. Each of us are sent into the world as an humble instrument to carry out God's spiritual providence by natural means; the Bible fully explains those truths, and nature has given capacity to every man to feel and know them. If we have sufficient sense to comprehend these sublime and spiritual truths, are we not equally able to understand our earthly and temporal ones?

Keills informs us, that in our bodies there are reckoned 245 bones and 446 muscles, for the purpose of motion; all these are ready every moment to perform their functions. It is supposed that 100 muscles at least are in constant action, for every breath we draw; we respire at least twenty times every minute; the heart beats in propelling the blood into the arteries from sixty to ninety times every minute, the stomach and muscles of the bowels are every moment in action; so that, without the least extravagance of expression, it may be truly said, that we enjoy 1000 blessings every minute. If we view all these countless blessings as we ought to do, and obey their laws, then we ought to feel grateful to him "whose hands have made and fashioned us," and who breathed into our nostrils the breath of life.

I have studied men, and I have found that they are always ready enough to understand their true interest, if it is presented clearly to their understanding; for when this is done, men begin to reason and reflect, and thus it may happen that what Archimides said of the mechanical powers of the lever, might be applied to the common-sense of man.

I contend, that if the simple science required for the study of nature's medicine were once instilled in young mind, he would by practical experience find, that nature had so constructed her work, as to be superior to all the ills or accidents to which man is subject; she gives them as she pleases, and by whatever rule she seems to us to scatter them for the use of mankind in every climate, that rule must remain a secret to man. As instruments, we have only the power to put the seed in the ground; but we do not know by what means the Almighty gives life to it; it is enough for us to know that such things are, and be thankful.

"For there are more things in heaven and earth
Than are dreamt of in our philosophy."
SHAKSPEARE.

Surely the higher classes should bestir themselves for their offspring, when they see, or at least ought to see, that the humbler classes of society are storing their children with useful knowledge - witness the extensive circulation of cheap literature. The common people of England are proudly disseminating useful practical knowledge over the surface of the globe, and practically exhibiting to mankind the inestimable blessings of the powers of the human mind.

I would not be considered an enemy to the highest systems of education; on the contrary, I sometimes think I might have been more useful had I not been so neglected in my own.

"I smile and say,
This is no flattery, these thoughts are counsellors
That feelingly persuade me what I am.
Sweet are the uses of adversity,
Which like the toad, ugly and venomous,
Wears yet a precious jewel in his head,
And this our life, exempt from public haunts,
Find tongues in trees, books in running streams,
Sermons in stones, and good in every thing."
SHAKSPEARE.

Every man, however humble his station in life, is endowed with a spiritual principle which he received by the "inspiration of the Almighty," whence result the faculties of consciousness, perception, memory, imagination, judgment, reason, moral feeling, &c. It is true, indeed, that there are great differences amongst men in the possession of those faculties; yet all excel in some one or more, sufficient to promote the end of raising them from a state of moral and intellectual degradation. We are all equal in the hope of immortality beyond the grave; all ranks must come to the same mortal termination— "Dust thou art, and unto dust thou shalt return." Again Proverbs xxii. verse 2nd; also Job xxxi, verse 15th; and Acts xvii. verse 26th. These quotations of the Bible contain not only a command for the practice of every virtue, but they also present us with some of the most striking and amiable examples of divine rule: "As ye would that men should do unto you, that do ye also unto them;" this precept runs through the whole of the Christian religion, and if my readers want to find a more explanatory account of all that constitutes the character of a just and happy man, let him read the 8th and 12th chapters of Romans, which contain most important advice, and recommend a practice of every thing that can render us amiable in the sight of God and man. These chapters, with proper reflections, ought to cause in our bosoms a universal love towards men of all nations, tribes, and ranks, as we are all children of the same Almighty Parent, and members of the same great family. Diversity of fortune and station appear absolutely necessary, in a world where moral evil exists; it is a wise and gracious appointment of the Creator, and is attended with many and important advantages, such as employing and putting to its proper use the several capacities and endowments of mankind, in those states of active exertion for which they are fitted, for their own good, and for the improvement and happiness of society in general.

To men of a contrary opinion (wishing to destroy and not improve), who think property ought to be equally divided and all men on a level, I have often observed, that the first law of God was order, which we can witness in all nature's works. We need go no further than the bee-hive: there will be seen the king, the queen, and every order of state down to the common labourers, who toil to collect the moisture from the foliage. These bees dare not enter the hive further than the spot marked out for them. Then there is another grade of bee, to take the load from them, and convey it to a sort of scaffolding; another bee of a superior order removes it to the roof, where the master bee is ready to plaster it on, precisely the same as a man does the ceiling of a room; while others of a superior class sit looking on, to see that each does his duty, and to administer comfort to the sick and weary, similar to the benevolent and charitable institutions surrounding us in this highly favoured country. In this faint and imperfect picture I have drawn, it will be seen that bees never work single, but always in companies, in the greatest order, that they may assist each other - *a useful hint to mankind*. By this judicious arrangement, the exertions of a single individual are rendered conducive to the ease, the convenience, the comfort, and the mental improvement of thousands. If all men faithfully performed their allotted task heartily, and contributed in their spheres to the prosperity and happiness of each, then the misery we every day witness would no longer walk "triumphant through the world," nor would the "world's laws" cause the widow and the fatherless to groan from the abuse of power, by those who have deprived them of comfort. The victims of seduction would no longer crowd our streets, but, instead thereof, purity, peace, and righteousness, would run through our world like a river, distributing safety, happiness, and repose. To dwell together in unity, to communicate useful knowledge, to teach each other, to assist the afflicted in every kindly office, and to prepare each other for that world which keeps this world in awe, should be the main business of life. The human mind, trained in wisdom, would be gradually prepared for entering on a higher scene of contemplation and enjoyment. What a happy world might this be if kindness and affection were the characteristics of the inhabitants thereof! and most fervently do I hope that, from the advance of science, and the improvement of education, this auspicious era may soon arise, when every comfort will be recognised as "coming down from the Father of Lights," and contemplated by enlightened understandings, with emotions of admiration and delight. On such a world the God of Heaven would look down with complacency, and his providential care would be exercised in averting those physical evils which have for many years been the punishment of the moral wretchedness of mankind, by the cunning artifice of man, by supporting the dogmas of mere quibbles and unmeaning ceremonies. Surely it is the height of ignorance to be attached to ancient customs, merely because they have existed, and do exist. In what situation will such stand at that solemn period when the present course of divine providence shall be completed on earth — when all the generations of men, both "rich and poor," being gathered together, will have to account for the deeds done in the flesh?

"In the corrupted currents of this world
Offence's gilded hand may shove by Justice,
And oft 'tis seen, the wicked prize itself
Buys out the law. But 'tis not so above
There is no shuffling — there the action lies
In its true nature, and we ourselves compell'd,
E'en to the teeth and forehead of our faults,
To give in evidence.
                    SHAKSPEARE.

Then it will be known if we have practised the very sweets of that religion, which says "Thou shalt love the Lord thy God with all thy heart, and with all thy soul, and with all thy strength." This is the first commandment; and the second very like unto it— "Thou shalt love thy neighbour as thyself." Every man, whether educated or uneducated, however humble his situation in life, however limited the gift of his knowledge, has it in his power to practise these two grateful affections, the first, to love his God; the second, to communicate blessings to his brethren.

"Are we not brethren?
So man and man should be;
But clay and clay differs in dignity,
Whose dust is both alike!"
                    SHAKSPEARE.

He can easily study Nature's laws, and also visit the sick bed of an afflicted neighbour; he can smooth his pillow, turn him round in his bed of suffering, and cheer him with expressions of tenderness and affection, and thus console his downcast spirit by his counsel and advice. I have proved, that *by* such friendly attentions, the mind has become so consoled, as, together with the use of simple means, Nature has cured the disease.

"From lowest place where virtuous things proceed,
The place is dignified by the doer's deed."
                    SHAKSPEARE.

God generally gives a blessing to proper means. He teaches the seedsman to sow his seed- who does not expect to reap wheat if he sows barley. So it is in the practice of physic; he that expects success, must first learn the cause of the disease, and then be conversant with fit remedies; when this is done, the rest must be left to the Almighty, whose moral as well as spiritual laws have never yet been brought into full effect.

" What is man,
If his chief good and profit of his time
Be but to sleep and feed? - a beast, no more.
Sure he, that made us with such power of comprehension,
Looking before, and after, gave us not
That capability and god-like reason

To mould in us unused."
SHAKSPEARE.

This is a subject from which we ought never to turn away - it lies fairly before us; the evil which requires our utmost industry to counteract. If all the energies and treasures that have been expended on an unjust war had been devoted in cultivating the principle of benevolence among men, this world would long ago have assumed a very different appearance to what it has for many years wore, through the enmity, malice, frenzy, and the unforiving disposition displayed by man towards his fellow; instead of bearing in mind that

"All souls that were, were forfeit once;
And *He*, that might the 'vantage best have took,
Found out the remedy: How would you be
If He, which is the summit of judgment, should
But judge you as you are? O, think on that,
And mercy then will breathe within your lips,
Like new-made man."
SHAKSPEARE.

I know that the majority of medical men will object to the young mind being medicinally educated, for reasons my readers will not want me to explain:

"That I remember now
I am in this earthly world, where to do harm
Is often laudable; to do good, sometimes
Accounted dangerous folly."
SHAKSPEARE.

I have long observed the times, and dispositions of men, and I think both are alike favourable to the supposition, that common sense, blended with honesty of intention, will ere long be universally in practice in the healing art, tending to the incalculable benefit of thousands who are now languishing in despair and hopeless misery.

"The image of it gives me content already,
And I trust it will grow to a most prosperous perfection."
SHAKSPEARE.

Such is the work we were sent to perform for each other. All the writings of St. James enjoin this; Paul approves of it; and He that came to save, who is no respecter of persons or sects, commands, when he says — "Inasmuch as ye have done this unto one of the least of these my brethren, ye have done it unto me." In order to carry this blessing into effect, it requires but a common-place understanding and talent. When the laws of Nature are studied by the repeated monitors she so often gives us of the cause and cure of disease, I am every day more convinced they must succeed, even after the failure of the splendid talents of the high flown college practitioner, whose science has carried him too far in the unnatural and dangerous mercurial kingdom. This opinion may raise the ire of some who would, for the sake of pounds shillings and pence, wish to support a mercurial practice; to such I would say -

"For shame! Be not offended,
I speak not in absolute fear of you;

I think our country sinks beneath the yoke!
It weeps-it bleeds; and each new day a gash
Is added to her wounds."

SHAKSPEARE.

The many applications that have been daily made to me by the Clergy, and by Charitable Institutions, since my first work appeared, to be instructed in *Nature's medicine* for the suffering poor, convince me that there is a ray of light rising on the mind of man in regard to the preventative and curative art. This science ought to be more open for social debate and improvement, than any other earthly thing that appertains to man, instead of being monopolized from age to age, by many who are not blest with sufficient sense to distinguish causes from effects. Can we have greater proofs of this wretched practice, than the many thousands of sufferers at this moment dying for the want of proper assistance to remove those juices which cause the disease? As far as my observation extends, I am of opinion that all pain proceeds from a stagnation of the impure juices of the body, which causes a compression of the membranes —the heart, the lungs, the liver, the kidneys, the flesh, the ligaments, the beautiful delicate fibres, the cartilage, the tendons, and above all the veins, arteries, and nerves; and as the stagnation and compression are greater or lesser, so is the pain. But the pain is different in parts, according to the difference of the membranes affected, for where there are the most nerves, there are the most sensations. Observe how every thing is arranged and tempered in this respect, to contribute to our comfort! The points of the fingers, which require to be possessed with a more delicate sensation than many other parts, are furnished with a corresponding number of nerves; at the heel of the foot they are more sparingly distributed, as it is required to be more callous. If those delicate feelings were equal over the whole body, our very clothes would become galling; and if every part were as insensible as the heel, the body would be benumbed, and we should lose the pleasure of that beautiful pliancy which infinite wisdom has designed for the active duties of life. When we consider how these delicate organs *are abused* in their uses, during a length of years, the only wonder to me is they last so long. If we consider the number of years those blessings are continued to us, if we count the number of nights we have passed in sound repose, the days we have enjoyed without pain, and from how many visible and invisible dangers we have escaped — when I, as an individual, think of those things, my thoughts are at once fixed into a melancholy, yet pleasing, and I trust not wholly useless reflection. He that feels that God is master of the actions of man, must not choose which part he will act, it only concerns him to be careful that what he is appointed to do, that he doeth it well.

I admit there have been discoveries made in the anatomy of the solids within the last fifty years, but I can find none made on the fluids of the body, wherein lurks the seat and cause of all diseases; these have been neglected, yet the profession abounds with men of such capacities, that if once they were to throw aside their college tuition, make experiments on the fluids, and let the humours be the foundation of their practice, they might act with some sort of certainty, to the great satisfaction and advantage to mankind. I may truly ascribe my success with my patients to having taken this view of the subject, and then finding some of nature's remedies to second and promote the natural efforts of the constitution to subdue and free itself from foul and noxious humours, which will sooner or later destroy the body and the mind. For an animated description of the evils here mentioned, see "Cases in Medicine by Wm. Stevenson, M.D.;" a work that no one of moderate understanding can read without deriving both pleasure and profit. Here will be seen the impropriety of making the Faculty the directors of the public mind. But I trust the time is not far distant when the usurped and unrestrained medical power over the minds of men will be entirely abolished; till then, I fear it is in vain to look for any great reformation in physic, and those who attempt it will have to contend with such a powerful and violent opposition, as must retard the progress of discoveries.

"To climb steep hills,
Requires slow pace at first."

SHAKSPEARE.

Let but a few in each town and village whom Providence has enriched with the gifts of independence, and made the treasurers of God's bounty, acting as the real guardians of the poor, find out and soothe the bed of sickness, bearing in mind that God provides his blessings to serve the needs of nature:

"Tis not enough to help the feeble up,
But to support him after."
SHAKSPEARE.

In this way clergymen, and charitable ladies and gentlemen, are doing more good in opposing and stopping the progress of disease with the assistance of a single well-contrived medicine, than is effected by the present practice of all the faculty within a hundred miles. I am of opinion that it would be a great improvement in the moral state of society if all the young clergy, both of the church and dissenters, were medicinally instructed; they would have ample opportunities of being useful in the sufferings of human nature. And such powers would rather increase the work of their spiritual visits than retard them; they could teach their patient to feel and know that all knowledge must be limited by religion, which at all times must be referred to for its action and use. Goodly actions, as well as preaching, comprise the duty of a clergyman; to comfort and relieve those who are on the bed of sickness, ought to be a great part of his employment:

" Be patient, for I will not let him stir,
Till I have used the approved means I have,
With wholesome syrups - drugs — and holy prayers,
To make of him a formal man again;
It is a branch and parcel of mine oath
A charitable duty of my order;
Therefore depart, and leave him here with me."
SHAKSPEARE.

So thought St. James, 2nd chapter, 15th & 16th verses: "If a brother or sister be naked, and destitute of daily food, and one of you say unto them, depart in peace, be ye warmed and filled, notwithstanding ye give them not those things which are needful to the body, what doth it profit?" In the prosecution of this noble end, man becomes "a worker together with God," an agent in carrying forward his plans of infinite benevolence, to the ultimate happiness of the universe. The moral and religious considerations to which I have now alluded, I have never seen taken into view by any medical writer, or in any address from the pulpit: yet it has often struck me that the miraculous powers given by our Saviour to his Apostles, chiefly fell within the province of medicine; all the Apostles in a certain sense might be considered as doctors. Could any other have written the 31st of Ecclesiasticus? Their powers, it is true, were extraordinary, yet they were principally exerted in the cure of bodily disease, and no doubt such benevolent acts had some tendency in gaining a footing for the doctrines their kind Master had sent them to preach.

When I review the conduct of the Deity, what provision he has made for the temporal comfort and individual happiness of man—when I reflect on what I every day witness, the anguish, the tears, the groans, and all the combined forms of wretchedness which are the attendants of accumulated diseases, such as

"A wretched soul - bruised with adversity,
We bid be quiet-when we hear it cry;
But were we burdened with like weight of pain,

As much - or more - we should ourselves complain."
SHAKSPEARE.

and when I witness the poor patient's deliverance from this bodily suffering, the mind then becoming softened, and, bursting with gratitude, his ear is open to the counsel of him who, as God's instrument, has effected his cure; this is the moment to drop the seeds of gospel truths, when earthly objects appear invested with their own soberness, and when they feel conscious that, through the singular mercy of God's restoring them to health, they may be brought into that state, that they will for ever relinquish the paths of vice, and become as a "man new made." Calling instantly upon God, he raises his supplicating hands towards heaven, and eyes bathed with repentant tears, to the Father of all mercies. Thus a once depraved mind, witnessing in his own person the manifest goodness of God, must have those feelings of delight and gratitude, which for ever after cause him to love his God and keep his commandments.

"Poor soul,
God's goodness hath been great to thee
Let never day nor night unhallowed pass,
But still remember what the Lord hath done."
SHAKSPEARE.

Opposed to the Lord, all power is weakness, supported by him, weakness becomes irresistible power; —and thankful am I that the eyes of the world begin to be opened, and the new doctrine I have recommended already gaining so much ground, that few authors or practitioners have in their own life seen the like to it. This unexpected encouragement has filled me with such a sense of gratitude, that I feel stimulated by an irresistible impulse onward in the work I have begun; and I doubt not, in spite of all the imperfections to be met with in my writings and practice, that many good and ingenious men will much improve on the hints I have here given.

"I to the world am like a drop of water,
That in the ocean seeks another drop."
SHAKSPEARE.

The christian-like charity to which I have here referred, I am happy to say, has for several years past been practised by many kind-hearted individuals. I will just give a few cases. Near Reading there lives a young clergyman only twenty-seven years of age, who, while at college studying for his profession, thought a little knowledge of medicine could do no harm. Soon after he was appointed to his present living my first publication was put into his hand; he entered so fully into my views that he determined on seeing me: when I instructed him in the use of my portable bath, and explained causes and their effects, and remedies for the same—advised him to go on in the good work he had begun, and advised him if he met with any difficulty, to write to me, and I would answer him without fee or reward. This he has done, and now this highly gifted young man, whose example is worthy the imitation of every person, is in full practice. To use the words of a neighbour "your pupil, the Rev. ******, may be seen travelling of a night from one sick house to another, giving, with his own hand, baths to the aged poor, and administering to them every comfort; he will soon starve the doctors, for he is curing all the diseases in the village." Oh, if such deeds were common, there would be no need of the cry, "the Church in Danger."

May he live
Longer than I have time to tell his years,
Ever beloved - and loving may his rule be;
And when Old Time shall lead him to his end,
Goodness and he will make up one monument."

SHAKSPEARE.

Another case is that of a most amiable young lady, the daughter of a country magistrate, who witnessed the cure I had performed on her beloved parent. Having told her the names of several herbs I had used, she begged me to supply her and she would attend to the poor in her neighbourhood. I did so, and when she wanted my humble advice she had it. The event will be seen in a letter from her father. He says:

"Your firm must be called Tilke and *******. My daughter must be considered a partner; with the means you sent, and the use of the spirit lamp, she is curing all the poor old ladies of dropsy and rheumatism, and she has such a high opinion of the holy thistle, that she desires as a favour you will furnish her with some of its seed, and with her own hands she will sow it in a piece of ground my gardener has marked out for her in my plantation; and she says it will be the most useful thing ever planted there."

Another young lady, who came to me a patient from Suffolk, had for six years been treated on the Abernethy system, and the action of mercury so long repeated had brought her to the very brink of the grave; no one thought she would have survived the first night she came into my house; I never witnessed any person in a more deplorable state from the destructive mercury. Delicacy alone prevents my giving particulars; suffice it to say, her bones were in such a state before she came to me, that almost the whole of the lower jaw -bone, together with the teeth, came away, entirely decayed. Her father commenced law proceedings against this injudicious practitioner — but the latter soon died, so the matter was never brought before the public.

This lady was in my house six weeks. In her first letter after she left me, she says, "I cannot find words to express to you my feelings for your skill and great kindness towards me during the the time I was under your roof; my friends were astonished to see me on my return. I am every day getting better." In a second letter she says, "I am quite well." I have this moment (1837) received a letter from her, wherein she says she never enjoyed better health; she left me in October, 1835.

This young lady has ever since devoted her time to the study of herbs, having the means, as well as a humane disposition. She is now willing to extend to others that knowledge which no doubt has been the means of snatching her from an untimely grave. In a letter in which she is asking my advice, and the properties of several herbs, she says, "I often envy your daughters the delight they must have in studying your charming pursuit; I am now so fond of it I could devote all my time to its cultivation and practice. The poor woman with the bad leg of years' standing I have nearly cured under your kind advice, and the means sent. You are not aware how highly I consider myself privileged in being allowed to refer to you, to assist me in my charitable work of curing the poor and needy. I am this moment going to visit a poor woman with a large family, who for a long time has been confined to her bed with rheumatism. I shall apply your little favourite camphor bath, and all other means in which you have instructed me, and have no doubt but that I shall succeed in the desired object."

This young lady, only about twenty-two years of age, sets a bright example to idlers and novel readers, shewing how useful every person may make themselves, however high their rank in society. In very select and similar cases, I am allowed to refer to the parents, and even the young lady herself. This reference, as a matter of course, is confined to females. The North River Times, published at Havershaw, tells of a young upstart of a doctor, recently settled in that village, who was a few days since called to visit a lady who had taken cold in a thumb from which she had extracted a thorn, and which had become inflamed. Young Bolus immediately administered fifty grains of calomel, and after watching the thumb with great anxiety for an hour, he prescribed a thumping dose of jalap, and went his way. In the course of the day he is again called, and had the satisfaction to find his patient enjoying a happy state of purgation, but still no alteration in the thumb: whereupon he sent for another round dose of calomel, and left her for the night. The lady, burning with an inwards fever, and unconscious of the nature of the drug she had taken, drank plentifully of cold water. Salivation ensued, and, though she saved her thumb, she lost her teeth, and, what is worse, her health is sacrificed for ever. The husband commenced a suit for damages: but the doctor proved that in all cases of this kind, the practice in question was according to Gunter - or in other words, was scientific; so that, in addition to the loss of his wife's teeth and health, the plaintiff lost his suit, and had to pay his own costs.

I will now introduce to my readers the case of a young lady and her aunt, who were fast falling sacrifices to the injurious effects of minerals; these fell in my way by mere accident, as will be seen. The wife of Dr.***** brought her two daughters to me with the Ringworn, and on each visit, while I was dressing their heads, she complained of her own dreadful sufferings, and what she had been told was the cause, namely, bile and the liver complaint; she had been told, and believed, that the liver was grown to her side, and all her friends thought she could not live long. Her looks told me what she had been taking, but she admitted that for two years her medical advisers (and such as are at the top of their profession) had been giving her calomel and blue pill to use her own words, "to scrape her liver." As she told me this tale, she saw me smile. She thus addressed me: "Mr. Tilke, whenever I am telling you my troubles you always smile - why do you do so?" My answer was, "If you were any other than the wife of Dr. ***** I would soon tell you; and what is more, I would almost as soon cure you; but I know that such prejudice must exist in the bosom of a man educated as your husband has been, and in those that are attending you, that all I could say or do would not be attended to." I then explained to her the cause—the effects her own feelings told her. I then said, if she would come to me for one fortnight (and her husband might come with her and see my practice), I had no doubt I could put her in that course of treatment, which would soon make her a strong woman." She went home and told her husband what I had said. The next morning for the first time he paid me a visit. I then explained to him, very fully my opinion. He at once proved himself a sensible man without prejudice; he placed his wife under my care, witnessed my practice, and slept in my house a fortnight. In two months she was in as good a state of health as ever she was in her life, and remains so up to the present moment, although four years have now elapsed.

Soon after I saw a niece of this lady, also the daughter of a professional man, but in a worse state than her aunt, as she had, from taking minerals, so stopt the efforts of nature, that all was wrong; she was nineteen years of age, and her beautiful features and form were changed to those of a *bloated person*. All desire for amusements was gone, and her mind impaired, so that she could not be left alone. Being the only child of doting parents, no expense was spared. By the desire of her medical attendants, her father took her to Paris, to try what the amusements of that gay city would do for her; horse exercise, and every thing that could be thought of, was tried, but all to no purpose. At last, when every hope was fled, her uncle and aunt (the doctor and his lady before spoken of) consulted me on the case, unknown to her parents. I at once pointed out to them where I thought the defect was, and the simple means nature had provided, to help, on the one hand, or to check on the other, that action of the body, which a wise Providence has ordained to the sex. I had an interview with the parents, and gave them hope I could save their afflicted child; the mother and daughter came, and in three weeks, with my baths and harmless herb tea, all was well.

Never, to the longest day of my life, shall I divest my ears of the sound of the convulsive sobs of the poor mother, when the functions of nature were once more regular. This amiable young lady has from that time (three years since) enjoyed the best of health.

The father and brother of the wife of the doctor before alluded to, afterwards placed themselves under my care. The father, (a captain in the navy), I soon cured, as I had nothing to do but work with my steam the mercury out of the system, strengthening and sweetening the blood with a decoction of holy thistle, comfrey, and flax. The son, an officer in the Indian army, was sent home an invalid, with the liver complaint. For a twelvemonth , although he saw what I had done for others in the family, he refused my assistance. At length he was in such a state, that I was fearful he was too far gone to recover. I made the attempt, and the medical gentleman who visited him almost every day, for the six weeks he was in my house, will feel pleasure at any time in stating what he saw of my practice. In three months, this gentleman was able to return to his regiment in the East- Indies. It will be seen I was truly successful in every case of this highly respectable family. I have given the particulars, as I believe that from very slight indisposition at first, the mineral practice, injudiciously applied, had aggravated to acute disease. I shall give one more case and then close the subject, feeling I have done my duty as an individual, in cautioning the public against its practice, and of substituting a simple and effectual remedy in its stead. A young gentleman aged twenty- three, son of a family of high rank, had for nearly two years been under a mineral treatment for a supposed liver complaint: at last it turned to what is very well understood in the medical profession, *A Mercurial Fever.*

> "Those of the raging fire of fever bred,
> And what's a fever but a fit of madness?
> But moody and dull melancholy,
> Kinsmen to grim and comfortless despair."
> SHAKSPEARE.

In this state he became my patient, and after he had taken about six baths, he found every morning on rising, a substance on his skin; he removed it by my desire and put it on a piece of writing paper; this was done for three or four days; he then showed it to a physician who was in the habit of calling at my house to visit one of my patients, who very candidly admitted it was a composition of quicksilver, which no doubt the patient's system was full of. This is only a case similar to many I have had. If any doubt this, by applying to me, I will refer them to where all doubt will cease. Having now endeavoured to show the cause, effects, and cure of indigestion, I think I cannot do better than close this subject, as I began, with a quotation from Shakspeare; and should I hereafter find that any thing I have here said has been the means of adding to the comfort of a fellow creature, my object will be attained, and I shall, in the full and happy hope of being useful, exclaim

> "O Thou, whose instrument I do account myself,
> Look on my doings with a gracious eye.
> To thee I do commend my watchful soul
> Ere I let fall the windows of mine eyes;
> Sleeping, and waking, O defend me still."
> SHAKSPEARE

It was my intention, in compliance with the wishes of my numerous patients, with whom I have been so successful in Dropsy and Scrofula in all its kinds, but more particularly in Scrofulous White Swelling, to have given my opinion of those two desperate diseases, my mode of cure, and their individual cases, for the good of the community at large. This I intended to do, and also to have written a *Medical Catechism* for the use of schools and private families, as I have had several masters of the former who have freely entered into my views of the universal good that may accrue to the young mind, morally and spiritually, (for both must work together,) by early being taught to know himself, and that man is not what, from his faculties, and the design of the Creator, he should be, in the relation in which he stands to the things of this world. When this be known, man will be free from those turbulent desires which keep him a stranger to himself, and the master will soon find out the boys that have a natural talent for the study of medicine. By causing such instruction, I might say,

> "Thus play I, in one person, many parts." -   SHAKSPEARE.

To such friends I have no other apology to offer for my non-compliance, than the want of physical strength, and being tied strictly down by my medical friends, (who I have long known have my interest at heart,) besides the intreaties of an affectionate wife, that I would not attempt it for the present. I am grieved to find the faculty of reason, or study, so much impaired from the great shock my poor body has suffered, that

   "Like a dull actor now,
   I have forgot my part, and I am out
   Even in all I knew." -   SHAKSPEARE

  Therefore I must be content to publish my opinion of Indigestion, and leave the subject of Dropsy and Scrofula for another season. I have been so blest in my attempt to cure those diseases, that I mourn my inability to complete the task I had undertaken. Did I say mourn! Oh no! for I consider every event "best as it is." My confidence is based on the 8th of Romans and 28th verse. Besides, morally speaking,

   "To mourn a mischief that is past and gone,
   Is the next way to draw new mischief on;
   The robbed, that smiles, steals something from the thief,
   He robs himself that spends a bootless grief."
         SHAKSPEARE.

  I am one of Nature's odd children, and always feel that my endeavours come very short of my natural desires for the public good. And what ever merit I have acquired for relieving my fellow creatures from pain, I have always wished that merit had been greater still, in order to show my self worthy of the gratitude and great respect that has been bestowed on me by every grade of society.

   "The friends thou hast, and their adoption tried,
   Grapple them to thy heart with hoops of steel."
         SHAKSPEARE.

   "Though I am satisfied, and need no more
   Than what I know, yet shall the oracle
   Give rest to the minds of others; and such as he,
   Whose ignorant credulity will not
   Come up to the truth."
         SHAKSPEARE.

  Nature's dictates tell me to do good when I can; this feeling prompts me even in dangerous cases to feel that

   "I dare do all that may become a man;
   Who dares do more, is none."
         SHAKSPEARE.

  The human mind was formed for different attainments and the accomplishment of some favourite pursuit, and the means whereby one endeavours to attain it, constitute the morality or the immorality of character. The school of adversity is the best to form a useful mind, and it appears essentially requisite, from the imperfection of our nature, that we must pass through great evil to attain great good. Our pursuits in the present life are frequently interrupted by disasters or dispensations, which throw a cloud on our prospects, and the most pleasing and prosperous circumstances of our affairs, for a season. But we always find pleasure, even in our prosperous days, to look back on the struggles we had to encounter in early life, and the hardships we surmounted by our own industry and perseverance. These virtues seldom fail to obtain a sufficient portion of wealth for all the wants of this life,

"For the world is but a shifting scene." - SHAKSPEARE.

I can truly say of myself that,

"There is a kind of character in my life,
That to the observer doth my history
Fully unfold; and it concerns me
To look into the bottom of my place
A power I have, but of what strength and nature
I am not yet instructed."
SHAKSPEARE.

I will not stop to discuss the question, whether the college practice or mine be right. I think life too short to spend our time in idle disputations; I am always ready to prove all I have advanced by practical facts. No doubt we both agree that

"By medicine life may be prolonged; yet Death
Will seize the doctor too."
SHAKSPEARE.

It is not the men that I find fault with, but the system of tuition and practice. No doubt the majority of the profession are, as I am, looking for useful knowledge—but God only knows which of us find it. It is unjust for ill-will to exist towards each other for our different opinions, which we cannot help; it is the man who acts wrong, and knows he does so, who is guilty, and not he who honestly and sincerely believes the wrong to be right.

I will give the different opinions of men, all of whom have been warmed by a college fire, on the subject of *Consumption*. No doubt each thought himself right, and that each considered his own remedies (although opposite to each other) effective. This bears me out in my opinion, that no man can prescribe a general remedy even for the same disease, upon all constitutions. Read what they say. One writer, *Stohid*, attributes the frequency of consumption to the introduction of Peruvian bark; another, *Morton*, considers the bark an effectual cure; a third, *Reid*, ascribes the frequency of the disease to the use of mercury; a fourth, *Brillonet*, asserts that it is only curable by this mineral; a fifth, *Rush*, says that consumption is an inflammatory disease, and should be treated by bleeding, purging, cooling medicines, and starvation; while a sixth, *Salvadori*, says it is a disease of debility, and should be treated by tonics, stimulating remedies, and generous diet. *Galen* recommended vinegar as the best preventative of consumption. *Desault* and others assert that consumption is often brought on by the common practice with young people of taking vinegar daily to prevent obesity. *Dr. Beddoes* recommended foxglove as a specific in consumption; and *Dr. Parr* found foxglove more injurious in his practice than beneficial. *Dr. Darwin* invented a dusting box for the application of powder to the surface of the lungs, for the cure of this disease; and *Dr. Fordyce, Johnston*, and others, attribute consumption in hair-dressers, stone-cutters, tailors, and knife-grinders, to the dust received into their lungs during respiration. These different opinions are, no doubt, intended by a wise provision of nature, to stir up men's minds to enquire and endeavour to find out the cause, why extremes and opposite opinions should all work, as it appears, against each other for the ultimate happiness of man. Nothing can be more opposed to each other than winter and summer, yet neither could exist for more than a season if it were not so. A man conversant with nature could spend a long life very usefully by writing on this subject alone.

I must now speak of myself, to explain to many of my old patients why I have not complied with their wishes, as many will only know of my inability to do so through the medium of this book.

Many of my observing friends have for several years past noticed, that by a perpetual exertion of the mind and body, my once naturally good constitution was fast giving way, and have advised me to give up my delightful study. Now, in a public point of view, my own feelings for some time have pointed out to me I cannot. No, if I were again to attempt it as I once did, I should lose all the purest pleasures of my mind, and in exchange for it I should feel debased and degraded by having been a traitor to those abilities, (which have proved useful though humble,) that God hath given me; and who has also supported me with courage to stand almost alone against such a powerful body, as my innovation could not but raise against me.

If my attentive readers refer to my opinion of the effect the mind has over the body, and learn the evils it has for many years produced on me by causing indigestion, they will suppose (and it is the fact) that I was splitting on the very rock I was guarding others against. To be brief, and I trust not tedious, I will give the case. For many months,

"Weakness possessed me and I was faint."
SHAKSPEARE.

Yet my anxiety and great flow of spirits kept me up; and on the 6th of December 1836, I completed my task on "Indigestion." Little did I think, when I concluded this subject with those beautiful words:

"To thee I do commend my watchful soul,
Sleeping and waking – O defend me still." - SHAKSPEARE.

I say, little did I think,

"To be so sad to -night
As this hath made me." - SHAKSPEARE.

or that in a few hours I should be in almost the agonies of death. At twelve o'clock that same night I was taken with violent spasms. Medical aid was called in, and every thing that human ingenuity could devise was tried from Monday until Saturday without the least relief. The whole of this time I had no sleep. My medical attendants began to think

" When remedies are past, the griefs are ended,
By seeing the worst, which late our hopes depended."
SHAKSPEARE.

They were of opinion on the Saturday that nature was nearly exhausted; yet still thought that

"Sleep, Nature's soft nurse," - SHAKSPEARE.

would rally me. But no: -

"In my heart there was a kind of fighting,
That would not let me sleep - methought, I lay
Worse than the mutinies in the Bilboes; rashly-
And praised be rashness for it -let us know,

Our indiscretions sometimes serve us well,
And that should teach us,
There is a divinity that shapes our ends,
Rough-hew them how we will." - SHAKSPEARE.

The soporific draught had no other effect than to cause most frightful visions of the brain, which appeared

"Sometimes like apes, that grin and chatter at me,
And often strike me; then like hedgehogs, which
Lay tumbling in my bare footway!
Like perspectives, which rightly gazed upon,
Shew nothing but confusion; eyed awry,
Distinguished form.
Filip me with a three man beetle;
With that, methought, a legion of foul fiends
Environed me, and howled in mine ears
Such hideous cries, that, with the very noise,
I trembling waked."
SHAKSPEARE.

It now appeared as though all would soon "be silence." Up to this time, one of my medical attendants, Mr. Joseph, had scarcely left me night or day: the other was immediately sent for. This was the moment when I felt, as I am sure they thought, that

"We cannot hold mortality's strong hand."
SHAKSPEARE.

Yet in this awful moment, I felt strong in the belief that

"There is a special providence in the fall of a sparrow -
If it be now, 'tis not to come; if it be not to come,
It will be now; if it be not now, yet it will come:
The readiness is all."
SHAKSPEARE.

Reduced as I was to the very last stage of existence, it has taught me a lesson I shall never forget, that the nearer the grave, the less the dread of "that country from which no traveller returns." When in health and prosperity, is the time to dread death, not in sickness, for then the world has lost every charm, and death every sting. There can be no doubt that this severe affliction was brought on from the power of sympathy, added to that of an overworking, both of the mind and body, the subject of Bile having absorbed my attention for the last twelve months. It must be understood that I cannot, from my engagements, devote more than one or two hours each day for writing; therefore my ideas press in upon me faster than my pen can record them. My mind being long fixed upon one subject, it gained such a predominancy over the body, that it is my belief, that the dripping of the biliary ducts into the bowels had for months ceased acting naturally; the consequence was, that the bile was thrown back in the reservoir or gall bladder, where it became petrified, and formed itself into gall stones. This is my opinion, although it may cause the unthinking to smile; but my object in stating this is, that it is worth the inquiry of those who wish to profit from causes, and their effects. Besides, I have a precedent to support this opinion. I once heard a paper read, "On the Influence of the Mind over the Body." The lecturer stated, that a friend of his had devoted years to the study of the formation of stone in the kidneys. When he had completed his task, he was taken with a spasmodic attack, and died in the greatest agony. On dissection, the cavities of the kidneys were found like a stone quarry; the stones were so large that they could not pass; and it was the opinion of all his friends that he died from intense study. Dr. Gregory and Mr. Joseph, in my case, both thought from the first it was a disease of the gall bladder, and the continual and violent spasmodic pains I suffered were a kind provision of nature sent to expel the gall-stones from the bladder, and pass them onwards into the bowels, similar, as they themselves said, to those pains felt by all Adam's daughters in the hour of nature's troubles.

Such affliction is a pill which, if wrapped up in dependence on Him who made all things perfect, may easily be swallowed, and the taste be as pleasant as honey in the mouth, or melody of music in the ear; but if discontent puts us upon chewing it, then it proves bitter and offensive.

Mysterious are the provisions of God to man, and when such afflicting visitations as these are sent us, submission and silence become our duty. The time was come when it was necessary to apply desperate means:

> "Diseases, desperate grown,
> By desperate application are relieved."
> > SHAKSPEARE.

They did so, and God blessed their endeavours, for in a few hours a great number of gall-stones passed. My pains left me, and, to the great joy of an affectionate wife and daughters, as well as that of my kind friends, they pronounced me out of danger.

Nothing that I can ever write or say, can express the high opinion I entertain of the professional abilities and judicious treatment I received in the hour of danger from Dr. Gregory, of Weymouth street, and Mr. Joseph, of Blandford street; and I am pleased, and I might add, proud to say, that a physician of very great eminence, on hearing of my illness, paid me a friendly visit. When he understood the means employed for my relief, and the two gentlemen under whose care I was, he said, he had so high an opinion of both, and so much approved of the treatment, that he could do nothing more than had been done to relieve me.

Although nearly a month has now elapsed since the attack, I do and must, for "a certain time," feel very weak, and am so much altered,

> "My face so thin,
> That in my bosom I durst not stick a rose,
> Lest men should say, look where the rushlight goes."
> > SHAKSPEARE.

If any conviction had been wanting of the gratitude and friendship of my patients towards me, I have had sufficient by the anxious and numerous enquiries from all classes during my painful and dangerous illness. The kind and feeling letters also received, deserve my most grateful acknowledgments, because they are from a class of persons born and brought up in a very different situation of life to that of my own. I will give one letter from a gentleman, a member of Jesus College, Cambridge, so humane and Christian-like, that I ought to be proud indeed at having the friendship of such a man. In a letter to my daughter, he says,

> "Dec. 10th, 1836.
> "It is with great concern that I learn by your letter of your father's illness; and I need not tell you, that beyond his own immediate family, there is not a person on earth has more sincere regard for him than I have; for independent of his skill and talent, and the gratitude I owe him for my recovery

from illness, I admire him for his moral and religious principles, and for his universal charity towards others.

"I wish I was as active as formerly, for then I should be at his bedside before this letter; but pray do not fail, if Dr. Gregory and Mr. Joseph have any doubt about his case, to call in the aid of some other person to a consultation on the subject; recollect he is public property, and of such a nature, that we cannot spare him without a great national loss being sustained. I was in the hope, when I last saw him, that his health had received great advantage from the journey he took: but I was equally aware that he was working too hard, both bodily and mentally. I dare say that Dr. Gregory and Mr. Joseph are right, about his disease being gall stones; still I cannot conceal from you, that although he is abstemious to a degree, yet it always appeared to me that there was in his constitution a tendency of blood to the head, and by his constant bodily exertions, added to those of his mind, he has called too much upon his brain, and that he requires to be more attentive to himself than he has been. He must not in future sit up all night writing, and making experiments; it is too much for any constitution to stand, however good it may originally have been. He must not in future, as regards his exertions, put on the full steam. Pray let me hear by return of post, and I should like to hear every other day. I pray that the Almighty may look down with pity and compassion upon him, and restore him soon to health, to his family, and friends. Give my most affectionate regards to him, and the same to yourself, mother and sister, and believe me to remain ever your sincere friend.

"PS.- I expect to be called to town soon, and my first visit shall be to Thayer-street. Why did you not write before? Send me full particulars what Mr. Joseph says about him; indeed, I hope he will find time in a day or two to write to me upon the subject, as I am so much interested about his patient."

According to his request, one of my medical attendants did write, and state all particulars; to which my kind patient wrote the following answer.

"Dec. 16th, 1836.

"In proportion to the grief I experienced from the first letter I received about my good friend Tilke's illness, so has my joy been at the account I have received from Miss Tilke's letter of Monday, and your's of this day, and I have to thank God, and you, for the very able, prompt, and decisive manner in which you treated his complaint, and for the present prospect of his perfect recovery. I well know how easily he is excited in his desire to cure his patients, and with how much enthusiasm he studies all complaints, and endeavours to find the remedy, and how anxious he is to reveal, in a great measure, the result of his discoveries for the benefit of the public; but if he wishes to do justice to himself and family, he must not be so enthusiastic — he must not put on the *full steam*; but must, till his health and strength is perfectly re-established, be more like his plan of making some of his medicines, which require to be *simmered for a long time,* in order to get out the virtues of the plants. Pray tell him from me, that I really beg of him to attend to your injunctions while he is your patient, as I did to him when I was his, and then he may hope to be sooner well than he will otherwise be if he neglects your advice and orders. He must re member his words to his own patients the moment they enter his house as patients: *they must obey his orders.* I return you many thanks for your satisfactory and explicit letter, and will thank you to express to your patient my delight at his being out of danger, and the hope that he will do his part towards his perfect recovery. With my kind regards to his family, and the same to yourself,

"Believe me to remain"

The advice given in both letters is "pure and honest," and such as I intend to follow. In this mournful description of myself, it will be seen I have given numerous quotations from Shakspeare, and must be allowed still to continue to do so. With me there is no study required to adopt Shakspeare's ideas, for they

"Come from my head as bird-lime does from holly."
SHAKSPEARE.

Still I cannot let the subject of Dropsy and Scrofula pass by without a few observations; and these, with a short correspondence (the transcribing of which I can entrust to a kind daughter) is all I dare venture on at this time. To those afflicted with the Dropsy, I can hold out a prospect of cure.

"They say miracles are past; hence it is,
That we make trifles of what were terrors."
                                        SHAKSPEARE.

To those who have been taught otherwise, I can only say,

"What I can do, can do no harm to try."
                                        SHAKSPEARE

To any one suffering under the Dropsy, and yet doubting of the chance of relief from me, I would say:

"He and his physicians are of a mind,
He, that they cannot help him,
They, that they cannot help.
How shall they credit a poor unlearned man,
When the schools embowelled of their doctrine,
Have left off the danger to itself!"
                                        SHAKSPEARE.

As I cannot, for reasons before given, go into particulars, I must insert one recipe that I have found do good in many cases, and cannot do harm in any constitution. Take

Half pint of dried Windsor Beans,
Two ounces of Green Dandelion Root,
Two ounces of Parsley Root,
One ounce of Ground Ivy;

boil this in one quart of water very gently for one hour, strain and drink this quantity every day. The beans ought to be put first in the water cold for one hour, before being put on the fire. This is a great diuretic, but a powerful astringent to the bowels, therefore the latter must be kept regular once or twice a day by taking

One ounce of Mountain Flax,
One ounce of Leaves of Senna,
Two ounces of Liquorice Root,

simmered in three pints of water for two hours. Take a wine glassful at a time. Should this treatment cause a fluid of an oily nature to rise up to the mouth, or by the bowels, it is a symptom of cure. I have never failed where this effect has been produced, caused, in my opinion, by the action of the beans. Continue this medicine for two months, and I can assure my readers from experience, that they will have no cause to regret taking my advice.

As to the Scrofula, I must of necessity be brief; it is that description of disease that Shakspeare himself was afflicted with, and the cause of his being lame for many years, and no doubt he spoke from experience when he said,

"Diseased nature oftentimes breaks forth,
In strange eruptions."—SHAKSPEARE.

I shall only give two cases, and these particularly by the desire of the patients themselves, as they were of the most desperate character. In this, like dropsy, I can hold out to the sufferer a prospect of cure. Those who think otherwise, I would say,

"I am not an impostor, that proclaim
Myself against the level of my aim,
But know I think, and think I know most sure,
My art is not past power, nor you past cure.
He that of greatest works is finisher,
Oft does them by the weakest minister;
It is not so with him that all things knows
As 'tis with us, that squares our guess by shows."
SHAKSPEARE.

The first case was that of a young man about eighteen. He was brought to me from Blackheath; his case was of that description commonly known by the name of a Scrofulous White Swelling in the knee, which was so bent that his foot came back almost to touch his hip. His case was so hopeless that I at once said to his uncle,
"This disease is beyond my practice."
SHAKSPEAKE.

He thought otherwise; and after much persuasion I consented to make a trial, on no other condition than that it should be under the daily inspection of a medical gentleman, as I thought he was too far gone for me to get my baths and medicine to act.

Extracts of letters from the patient and his cousin will shew the happy result. He says,

" Had not Providence led my friends to consult you, I must either have lost my leg or my life, if we refer to the opinion of the three medical gentlemen who examined me, and stated that "I must have my leg amputated, as it was perished". In three weeks after they stated this, I could walk without a stick; I am now in perfect health."

His cousin writes as follows:

"Dear Sir, –I desire to acknowledge with gratitude your very great care and attention to my cousin; and, on reflection, I can but admire the guidance of Providence that he was brought to you. His case being considered acute rheumatism by the medical gentlemen who attended him, and we, knowing your skill in the curing of that disease, placed him under your care in December 1833; you immediately discovered that it was not rheumatism, but, what was far worse, a deranged state of the bodily system, and a decided white swelling in the right knee. He was an inmate of your house three weeks, during which time the kindness of Mrs. Tilke and yourself was truly parental. He then returned home, and you assured us, if we paid attention to what you prescribed, that his knee would again become perfect. I implicitly followed your rules, and with delight I saw his health improve daily. For the satisfaction of our friends I took him to -(blank); there were three medical gentlemen present, who told me, as soon as they saw the knee, 'that they could do nothing for him, as the leg was perished, and that it must come off, and the sooner the better.' To my great joy, in less than a month he was able to walk without a stick. On the 3rd of March he again commenced his occupation, which he has pursued ever since; he does not walk the least lame, nor find any inconvenience from the disease he has had. It is not unlikely that this may appear to some whose eye it may meet to be an exaggerated statement; but I shall feel most happy at any time to bear personal testimony to the facts here stated. Sincerely hoping that success may still attend you,

"I am yours, ever grateful,

"E. A. "

While this youth was under my care, a gentleman of high standing in the profession, residing near Piccadilly, (who allows me the honour of referring to him to prove this case) was in the daily habit of visiting a patient of mine, who had been under his care for several years. I succeeded so much to his satisfaction, that he asked me to let him know when I had any difficult case, and he would call and witness the cure. I sent for him to see this youth; he at once pronounced it White Swelling, and in that stage he thought incurable. Family affairs took this gentleman into the country for a fortnight: on his return he called to see my patient, and was surprised to find he was gone; and when I told him he could walk, he said, "Tilke, I have that opinion of your veracity, that I would believe anything you told me for a truth; but I have stated his case to a medical friend, and told him I should watch your treatment; but if I tell him what you have just stated, without seeing the lad, why I should be laughed at." My answer was, "Sir, invite your friend to your house any day you please, and I am sure my young patient is so grateful, that to oblige me he will come to town and visit your own house." He did so, and the knee was examined: when this kind and generous man gave a sort of lecture on the case, urging the propriety you of never removing a limb until every other means had been tried, and pointing out the necessity of perseverence in the profession. "You, young man, said he, "have to thank Mr. Tilke for having two legs to walk upon instead of one." Although I became this gentleman's successful medical rival in one case, he acted thus liberally towards me, and up to the present moment I have the honour of enjoying his friendship.

In a letter to another person, who afterwards became my patient, he says, "I would recommend you to try Mr. Tilke; he is not a regularly educated medical man, but he is a clever one, and what is above all, an HONEST ONE." This, Shakspeare goes, says, as the world goes

"Is to be one man picked out of ten thousand."

"If," he continued, " he thinks he cannot cure you, he will say so. You are perfectly safe in trying him, as he exercises so much judgment in his treatment, and the means he uses are so simple that he cannot hurt you."

And it should be observed, that this patient was recommended to me by this gentleman, entirely without my knowledge.

"Look on this picture, and on this! "

mentioned in pp. 172, 173, of the second edition, in this book; here my readers will see the counterfeit presentment of two college practitioners. To that liberal and kind man, who has done so much to encourage me, I can only say,

"My kind Sir, I can no other answer make,
But thanks, and thanks, and ever thanks,
Often good turns are shuffled off, which such
Uncurrent pay: but, were my worth,
As are my feelings, firm, you should
Find better dealing.
I have a desire to hold my
Acquaintance with you, or rather my
Knowledge, that I may say hereafter

He is a just man I know."
SHAKSPEARE.

As to the conduct of the person, mentioned in p. 172 of this book, I will not trust myself to say all I feel; for "since my poor heart knew itself," I have always despised an illiberal man. It is this unwarrantable conduct that

" Blurs the grace and blush of modesty,
Calls virtue hypocrite; takes off the rose from the fair
Forehead of an innocent love, and sets a galling blister there.
SHAKSPEARE.

This weak man was then in the very prime and vain pride of his glory; but now he is

"Not where he eats, but where he is eaten;
A certain convocation of politic worms are even at him now.
We fat all creatures, to fat us, and we fat ourselves
For maggots. Humph — this man might be in his time
A great buyer of land, with his statutes, his recognizances,
His fines, his double vouchers - is this the fine of his fines
And the recovery of his recoveries, to have his fine proud
Pate, full of fine dirt!"
SHAKSPEARE.

My object in stating this, is like the directing post, to prevent our going the wrong way by envious feelings, instead of cultivating good-will towards each other. I trust that my readers will feel

"That my disclaiming from a purposed evil
Frees me so far in their most generous thoughts,
That I have shot my arrow over the house,
And hurt my brother."
SHAKSPEARE.

I forgive him, by the same rule as I hope to be forgiven.

The next case is that of a young gentleman afflicted with that description of scrofula known by the name of Leprosy. This was also shewn to another medical gentleman, who can prove that the ulcers were so deep, that by probing, I could touch the bone. I give the patient's own letter, written two years after the cure. I have likewise the privilege, in select cases, of referring to him personally.

"Oct. 29th 1836

"Dear Sir,—Having understood that you were about compiling a new work on your system of treating various diseases, I take the opportunity of now publicly returning my sincere and heartfelt thanks for the almost miraculous cure which, through the aid of Divine Providence, you have performed on me, by your simple though effective method. If you should think it worth while to make any use of this communication, I will state my case as briefly as possible, for the benefit of those who may have suffered from the same causes as severely as myself, in the full hope that it may be the means of dispensing your talents and exertions in a more extended sphere. Being naturally of a very scorbutic habit of body, at any time I took cold I always had a rash appear on the back of my hand, the inside of the thighs, and all over my legs. Unfortunately I caught a severe cold during last September twelvemonth, which settled in my system, and affected the parts before-mentioned to that degree, that I was literally one mass of ulcers, accompanied by the formation of a very bad abcess on the thickest part of the thigh, near the hip joint, for which I was under the necessity of being twice operated upon; and after suffering a martyrdom under the treatment of my surgical adviser, (who was a very dear friend,) I was recommended to you, I might truly say in the eleventh hour — and, to the astonishment of myself, and the joy of a dear mother and friends, I was so much recovered, that in eighteen days from the time I was placed under your care, I was able as usual to attend to my business. I am now, and have been ever since, in the enjoyment of the most perfect health, and have never had the least sign of a return of the old disease. If I was to write till doomsday, I should never be able sufficiently to express my gratitude for your kindness to me while a patient; and the very kind treatment I have uniformly met with from yourself and family since that time, will never be obliterated from the memory of, dear Sir,

"Your most obedient and much obliged servant,
"J. W."

These diseases are of so complicated a nature, that, without going into the particulars of the different effects produced on each individual, I can not give the different remedies that I apply ; but for the present must content myself by giving one which can do no harm, but real good. Take

Four ounces of Red Dock,
One ditto Dandelion,
One ditto Holy Thistle,
Two ditto Ground Ivy;

Boil this in three quarts of water till reduced to three pints, drink one pint every day. Should this not act on the bowels, keep them regular by taking

One ounce of Lenitive Electuary,
One ditto of Milk of Sulphur,
One ditto of Cream of Tartar.

Should the sores be very painful, use an ointment made from goose-grass and fig leaf, spoken of in this work.

I must now say a few words on the subject of Gout, as I have promised several friends that I would publish their letters; and although I have had for seven years a constant, and I might say the largest practice of any man living, I have seen no thing to alter the opinion I first formed of this disease. Of course, experience has taught me how to apply means best suited for different constitutions.

The following letter is from a gentleman who was given up by his medical advisers as incurable, in consequence of a tendency to dropsy and erysipelas attending his gout. This letter has been given up to me by an honourable Baronet, who has for many years taken much interest in my practice, and who himself received it from my patient.

"April 9th, 1836.

"My Dear Sir- I hope this letter will be more successful than my last, which followed you half over England. I thank you for your kind inquiries after my health, and am happy to say it was never better in my life. Yet this damp weather prevents me getting so strong in my knees as I could wish; however, when settled weather arrives, I expect to gain my usual strength. When I consider what I suffered for nearly two years, with confinement to my bed with the rheumatic gout, and all the medical men whom I consulted, together with the aid of ****** (sic), did not give me any relief, but, on the contrary, I grew worse, I have great reason to be thankful that I was prodentially and accidentally led to place myself under Mr. Tilke. Nothing that I can say will express to you how highly I consider his talents as relates to those cases which have been hitherto considered incurable, but most of which, if not all, have given way under his treatment; and as it regards gout and rheumatism, he seems really to play with them, so certainly and so expeditiously does he conquer the disease entirely, and eradicate it out of the constitution, of however long standing it may have been; and in common cases of gout he appears to cure it in a fortnight. Of course, where it is constitutional and has been long in the system, and where the medical men have been driving it into the constitution by colchicum, or the eau medicinale, instead of forcing it out of the constitution by baths, and by purifying the blood, the cure will require more time in proportion to the time it has been in the system, and merely checked, but never eradicated.

"Whenever I now see a friend of mine afflicted with the gout, I say to him, 'Mr. Tilke can cure you, and if you will not go to him I shall not in future pity you.'

"I shall be in town soon, and shall hope to see you.

"I am, my dear Sir -

"Yours, most truly, &c."

The next letter is from a scientific gentleman, as his kind and ingenuous letter will imply.

"Dec. 11th, 1835.

"Dear Sir,-Agreeably to my promise and your request, I write to inform you of the good or bad success which has followed the mode of treatment laid down by you for me to pursue, to effect a cure of the gout. I had scarcely need say, I adhered most scrupulously to it, and to my great delight, found it highly efficacious. I have experienced only one paroxysm since I became your patient, and that of so mild a nature and of so short duration that it could hardly be denominated gout; it was not of that description which Dr. Johnson calls 'the eighth plague', but what is termed in the phraseology of gouty subjects, 'a slight touch'.

"I await, anxiously await, the arrival of the day on which I am to return to your hospitable roof, to be metamorphosed into a joint, for the purpose of annihilating that destroyer of my happiness and producer of all my woe — the gout. Well may Dr. Johnson say, 'the eighth plague is the gout,' and 'that man,' continued the learned lexicographer, 'who discovers a medicine to alleviate its torments deserves well of his country; but he who can effect cure should have a monument raised to his memory as high as St. Paul's, as wide as the Thames, and as lasting as eternity.' God grant I may, at no distant period, receive such demonstrable proofs in my own person, as to justify me in publishing to the world, that Mr. Tilke is the individual entitled to this colossan monument of national gratitude.

"My best wishes and compliments attend Mrs. Tilke and family, and believe me,

'Dear Sir,
                Yours, sincerely."

"PS. Since writing the above, I have felt those symptoms which indicate the near approach of a fit; but I hope for the best, and console myself with a firm belief in your skill, when you shall be afforded an opportunity to exercise it on me, to receive those benefits which I firmly believe no other person but yourself can confer."

The following is from a scientific botanist and mineralogist, who has travelled perhaps a greater distance, and made a larger Botanical collection than any man living. I feel the greater desire that this gentleman's letters should be given in full, as the approbation of one who has studied botany scientifically must be of the greatest importance to myself, at the same time that it must appear to my readers the strongest corroboration of what I have advanced in these pages in favour of Vegetable Medicine.

"Feb. 1837.

"Dear Sir,—I learn you are about to publish another edition of your work, and also with additional information upon Indigestion and Bilious Complaints. I do not write this letter to you in the hope of your getting any additional patients - on the contrary, after your late illness I am anxious that you should not have so much exertion of body and mind. Yet I much wish that it may assist you by bringing forward your system into general notice, and I am still sanguine that your work will meet the eye of some person of rank and wealth, having the disposition to do good to his fellow creatures, and who may be induced to come forward and patronize the erection of a Hospital, where your system of cure may be introduced under your superintendence, and then I have no doubt that several well educated young men intended for the profession will enlist under your guidance, and will perform many cures that are now considered by the profession incurable; and I will venture to predict that, with attention, those young men will far outstrip those of the same standing, both in practical knowledge and pecuniary profit. I am perfectly satisfied, if this plan is properly brought forward, there is not, among the many patients whom you have cured, one who would not cheerfully and anxiously join it with donations and annual subscriptions, according to their means - and none more so than myself.

"I will not enumerate the many successful cures that I have witnessed performed by you of Ringworm, Scrofula, Leprosy, &c. &c., many of which are, even now, considered incurable; but you may refer any sceptics to me, and I could soon convince them of your success. I have not mentioned *Gout* above, as I consider you would never fail in curing that in any person under sixty years of age, how ever long he may have been subject to it.

"Wishing you health and prosperity, believe me,

Your sincere friend,

"AMICUS."

The gratitude and kindness of this gentleman for my humble though successful efforts in the restoration of his health, have no limits. With many other kind presents, on his birth-day he sent me a book, containing an account of the medicinal properties of nearly eleven thousand plants. No one would conceive the value this book is of to me. It has been printed two hundred years, and even then it could not have been bought for less than thirty guineas: now, that such a work is scarce to get, it is worth double that sum.

This volume is a proof, at once, of all I have advanced,that Nature has provided bountifully, but that Man has been ungratefully negligent. I find much in this rare work corroborating what I have long said on the astonishing properties of many herbs and roots with which I was already familiar; and an immense fund of information beyond what I could have gained, perhaps, in any other work. The kind donor wrote in the book the following:

"To Samuel Westcote Tilke,
 "8, Thayer-Street,
  " Manchester Square.

"Although this book, containing the medicinal virtues of several thousands of plants, has been published two hundred years, yet it was not till 1830 that the British public derived the full benefit of the work in curing disease. At that period, a person who had for several years observed the increase of diseases, and the general neglect in the cure of them by vegetables, began by voluntarily and charitably *curing the poor* of that troublesome complaint the Ringworm. Having succeeded in this in every instance where the attempt was made, he was determined to apply his mind to the study of the healing and beneficial effects of vegetables, instead of minerals and poisons, so generally then made use of by the medical profession. By frequent experiments, he found that the rheumatic gout, leprosy, scrofula, dropsy, and cancerous complaints gave way to his remedies, aided by his medicated vapour baths The fame of these cures being communicated by the relieved, the applications from all ranks became so numerous, and interrupted his business so much, that it became absolutely necessary for him to give up his trade, and to take a house for the express purpose of curing these several hitherto considered incurable diseases. This celebrated person is the above -named Samuel Westcote Tilke; and I have reason to be grateful to him for my cure, and feel that I can never adequately pay him for the benefits derived. By way of encouragement (if it were wanted), I conclude with the following quotations

"He that hath pity on the poor, lendeth unto the Lord; and that which he hath given, will he pay him again.' Prov. xix. 17.

"Blessed is he that considereth the poor and needy; the Lord will deliver him in the time of trouble.
"TheLord will preserve him and keep him alive, and he shall be blessed upon the earth, and thou wilt not deliver him unto the will of his enemies.

"The Lord will strengthen him upon the bed of languishing; Thou wilt make all his bed in his sickness.' Psalm xli. v. 1, 2, 3.

"Nor can I conclude this without remarking, when I read the 112th Psalm, how forcibly I am reminded of Mr. Tilke's character."

With this valuable present I received the following letter.

March 1st, 1836.

"My Dear Sir, - I beg your acceptance of the accompanying volume of 'Gerard's Herbal,' which was published two hundred years since, and never appreciated as it ought to have been by the profession of medicine. You alone seem to have practised healing and curing divers diseases by the most simple herbs, and you are therefore more worthy of this book than any other person; and it will be a great consolation to me, if hereafter I shall learn that you have derived any valuable information from the perusal of it. I had great difficulty in getting the bookbinder to finish it soon enough to send it you on my birthday, as a birthday present. Believe me to remain, dear Sir,

 "Your most grateful and sincere friend."

On the same day I wrote the following answer:-

" My dear Sir,—Had you consulted Shakspeare, he would have told you, that it was

"Cruelty to load a fallen man."

I mean this in a spiritual, as well as a moral sense. We are so apt to forget our duty to God and man, when such prosperity as I am now experiencing overtakes us. You my dear sir, who have been

"Tried and tutored in the world,"
SHAKSPEARE.

ought rather to guard and caution me against self ambition, and that ignorant pride, which arises from the vain and wicked heart: for in that valuable present which you have made me of 'Gerard's Herbal,' you have, from the best of motives no doubt, without the aid of pencil, drawn me in that character which I can never assume. To an unlettered man like me it is dangerous, for

" There may be in that cup
A spider steeped, and one may drink - depart,
And yet partake no venom - for his knowledge
Is not infected: but if one present, make known
How he hath drank, he cracks his gorge, his sides
With violent heavings."
SHAKSPEARE.

"But I think you suppose, what is the fact, that

"I will frown, and be at enmity
With cozening hope; he is a flatterer,
A parisite, a keeper back of death,
Who gently would dissolve the bands of life;
Which false hope lingers in extremity. "
SHAKSPEARE

"O, sir, if I had the credulity to be vain, from the whispers and letters of praise that I daily hear and receive, I should be a lost man indeed. Why should I be proud for having to exercise that knowledge, which is only lent me? for

" Nothing can we call our own, but death,
And that small model of the barren earth
Which serves as paste and cover to our bones."
SHAKSPEARE.

"However, I will forgive you this time, if you will promise to do so no more. I am sure you will be pleased to find that the dangerous parts of the effusion of praise fell on me

"Like water in a sieve." -   SHAKSPEARE.

"But yet I cannot but appreciate in its proper sense, and forcibly feel the very great kindness of your invaluable present, and the kind and friendly manner you have been pleased to speak of me. I trust no act of my future life will ever make you blush for having formed so favourable an opinion of so humble an individual, who has felt

"How difficult it is to do good,
While to do wrong is so easy."
                                    SHAKSPEARE.

for seeing, as I must see, or ought to see

"'Tis the great art of life
To manage well
The restless mind;"
                                    SHAKSPEARE.

for having been a slave to the influence of my own opinions, early acquired, and carrying the same into effect for the benefit of my fellow man, always despising the idle reasonings of speculation, on a science where facts alone should hold the sway. No one is more indulgent than I am as regards the common weakness of human nature; but when I see the medical practice become really criminal, and the depravity of the licentiates of the present day, —when I see truth and common sense dwindle away, and scarce any of the virtues which adorned and signalized our ancestors remain, -I say this is enough to make one feel and exclaim, that he is the benefactor to mankind who discovers the virtues of medicinal herbs, and applies them to the relief of the afflicted; --a pleasing office, ever grateful to a benevolent mind. If I have shown any wisdom by a judicious application of them to the cure of diseases, what must that wisdom be which gave them their forms and properties, which work so easily together! And being ordained with so much apparent foresight, can we for a moment hesitate to determine whether they are the effects of chance, or the providence of a merciful God, who has given us vegetable medicine for every season of the year, incidental to our maladies. It was these feelings that aroused me, and brought me forth as a public man, in the station of life in which Providence hath now placed me. When I heard the word incurable, and that too coming from medical men, 'For shame,' said I, 'it is a disgrace to the dignity of the medical profession.' I then thought the word must arise from either a wicked, or a very ignorant mind; if it was so either way, it was wrong, for they as practitioners ought to feel and know this simple truth, that for every disease there is provided an antidote. A slight inquiry into the laws of nature, will satisfy any reasonable and rational being of this fact; and I am a proof that it requires but a common understanding to carry this blessing into effect: for knowledge is like virtue, it consists of an humble opinion of our own abilities, and we gain strength in becoming sensible of our weakness. This feeling has taught me to pursue the road which nature has pointed out for man to take. In this enquiry, I have found easy observations, useful discoveries, enjoyments of every sort, without instruments, without books, or even without education. Man as yet has but faint perceptions of the boundless field of nature; it surpasses all the efforts of the mind. I have had but slender means of proving this, but yet a day has not passed without some agreeable discovery being added to my stock, and establishing in me the limited share of physical knowledge which I possess. Then to put this in practice, I keenly and sensibly felt the high and responsible situation in which I stood; that the life, the health, the happiness, and comfort of thousands, might in a great degree depend on my advice, information, and bodily exertion; and having, previous to this, perused the volumes of Shakspeare, to pick up in my own way, little odds and ends of information, as to the manner and treatment of diseases by our ancestors, I gained a correct conception (as I think) of causes, and their effects, acting on the mind and the body, explaining every thing that is closely connected with the healing of the one, and administering of comfort to the other. But I thought of his words,

"If we should fail !" - SHAKSPEARE.

Yet, again he says,

"But screw your courage to the sticking place
And we'll not fail."

"The sense of these words is perfectly evident; and mean, brace up your resolution so firmly, as not to be always wavering and slipping back, but take courage, and stick to the resolutions that you have formed in any station of life, but more particularly in dispensing God's blessings to man, and establishing its reputation beyond the possibility of doubt. Yet how carefully has he shewn the wisdom of the Creator in denying to man a knowledge of futurity; he says,

"If one might read the book of fate,
And see the revolution of the times,
How changes fill the cup of alteration
With divers liquors! O, if this were seen,
The happiest youth, viewing his progress, through
What perils past, what crosses yet to come;
Would shut the book, and sit him down and die."
SHAKSPEARE.

"He shews us easily the course of study best adapted for man, to know himself; he shews us, as far as human sagacity has penetrated, all that is known concerning the Deity; he opens to us all that is existing in nature, that should qualify a man for that particular occupation which Dame Nature hath appointed him to fill; he supplies him with means to remove obstructions, he presents him with supplies to enable him to prosecute his designs with vigour and success: he tells us that the present moment we may call our own, but the next is at the disposal of God - here is a solemn reflection, big with importance, making a most striking appeal to the conscience of every one who is unconcerned and indifferent, as regards the affairs of the immortal soul. He says,

"Fools that we are,
Never to think of death and of ourselves
At the same time, as if to learn to die
Were no concern of ours! 0, more than sottish,
For creatures of a day, in gamesome mood,
To frolic on eternity's dread brink,
Unapprehensive, when, for aught we know,
The very first swoln surge shall sweep us in."

"O that we all could feel these words in the sense Shakspeare intended them! Not to leave repentance until our wits are distracted, the understanding gone, our bodies harassed and tormented with the throbs and pains of mortal sickness; not to leave those awful matters, and strive to become sudden saints when we are scarce able to behave ourselves like reasonable creatures; who only cease to offend their Maker, when the ability of offending is taken from them.

You say the works of 'Gerard' have not as yet been fully appreciated. This I fully grant, and at the same time think that the beauties of Shakspeare are as yet scarcely known, for it was he who taught me first to inquire into the sheet anchor of my practice - namely, the holy thistle, the sage, the rue, the balm, the wood betony, and many others others; it was he who pointed out this singular fact, that if any plant is drooping or dying, place a plant of camomile near it, and it will recover; it was he who discovered that rue and sweet basil would not grow together, or even near each other. You, "no doubt, as a scientific botanist, may easily explain those wonders of nature to mankind; you have the ability and the time, I have neither; you have a fine scope to show the 'mirror up to nature.'
"Again thanking you most cordially for your useful present, may you, my dear sir, live long to enjoy the society of your happy family, and that

"Good digestion wait on appetite,
And health to both,"

is the sincere wish of your grateful friend ,
"S. W. TILKE."

The insertion of this correspondence may appear like egotism on my part, to those who do not know me; but I can assure them it is done at the particular desire of many sincere friends, as it explains exactly the position of life I stand in with the public, better than any account I have before given. I am grateful to them all for their kind feelings towards me; but there is a power to which I look up with a thankful heart for the manifold blessings and kind provision for my prosperity and usefulness. The daily blessings to us all are beyond our comprehension. If we feel disposed to be grateful for mercies already received, where shall we begin? What man can conceive the loving kindness of Him whose tender mercies are over all his works! It is no small mercy, that we are allowed to enter this present year, when we reflect that nearly forty millions of our suffering fellow creatures must have died in the year that has just ended; and of this great number it is awful to think how many have ceased their earthly pilgrimage,
"With all their imperfections on their head!"
SHAKSPEARE.

We must not despair; we know that God's ways and ours are not alike - even in this world, we must trust to his loving kindness, that he has provided a way peculiar to himself to pardon sin; if not, few can ever reach that happy mansion, spoken of in the 14th chapter of John. How different are the promises held out by him in this chapter, who became poor and suffered for us; to the threat held out to sinners in the 18th chapter of Ezekiel and 20th verse, where it says, "the soul that sins shall die," that is, shall suffer punishment. I have drawn my readers' attention most seriously to the cure of the body, that only lives for a short time; I cannot conclude this subject without calling most earnestly their sincere attention to the care of that soul, that must live in eternity, either in bliss or misery.

"Let us go to our bosom,
Knock there, and ask our heart what it doth know."
SHAKSPEARE.

Let us look within and read it there; read it in the troubles, the remorse, the forebodings of our own conscience. Why are we uneasy, when any thing reminds us of the approach of Deity? why has sickness, or sudden death, or viewing an open grave - why have such sights and thoughts power to alarm us? The answer will be plain, because we have "left undone the things we ought to have done; and have done those things which we ought not to have done, and there is no help in us;" unless intercession is made for us through Him who came to save. If we feel and believe all this, and go on still displeasing God, where is our gratitude to him? Speaking as a poor mortal man, I can say, that nothing is so cutting to me in this life as ingratitude; if these be the feelings of men in general (which I believe), what must be those of God, who has already made such sacrifices for us, and prepared a place for the good and happy? But when men continue in their wicked course, conscience is ever tender, scrupulous, and fearful; they are soon terrified, and always looking for the punishment they have so justly deserved. Man is a rational being, but with cunning sufficient to give all his actions the colour of reason. What he cannot forbear, he will endeavour to justify; what he cannot justify, he will extenuate; and what he cannot extenuate, he will endeavour to excuse, and raise up "Mammon" of his own begetting, which will represent money ill gotten, profit unworthy, fraud, scheming, hard - heartedness, hatred of the poor, contempt for misfortune, and every odious attribute that can dishonour human nature. I would ask those who are in the habit of attending the sick and dying, if they have not often witnessed such expressions of contrition for deeds done, by those who have

> "Been struck so to the very soul,
> That presently they have proclaimed
> Their malefactions."

For such deeds,

> "Though it hath no tongue,
> Will speak - with most miraculous
> Organs to the guilty mind."
>   SHAKSPEARE.

I trust that there are but few such men to be found , and those, I would advise to lose no time in accomplishing the "consummuation so devoutly to be wished," that of being happy in this life, and in a prospect of future felicity. This can only be accomplished by being good and doing good; it behoves every man who is accountable to his God for all his actions, that when he is about to accomplish any important affair, he should retire alone, and ask his own heart: If I do this act today, will it make me unhappy tomorrow?-would it make my pillow hard if I was on my death - bed? There is a little *Cherub* in that heart, that will tell him if it be wrong, when he at once ought to say — to gain the "whole world," I would not do it. But, for the want of this self- examination, many a naturally good-disposed man

> "Can accuse him of such deeds,
> That it were better his mother had not borne him."
>   SHAKSPEARE

While I am endeavouring to urge a subject so important, let me entreat my readers to employ their minds, not in determining the awful condition of others, but in judging of their own:

> "Let every man prove his own work."

I have done so as an individual in the scale of self-examination, and am found much wanting:- I blush when I state, that on reference to my Journal of 1810, I find I am not so good a Christian as I was at the age of sixteen. Year after year I have promised to amend; time has been spared me for this purpose: I once thought, that when I was comfortably settled in the world, I would begin; when this comfort was attained, my excuse was, when I had attained a sufficiency. This I fear is the excuse of many. To my disobedience in my duty to God, I plead guilty ;—but if accused of not performing my duty to my fellow-man, I plead not guilty. I am a slave to that feeling, which already has given me that inward comfort which no man can take from me. To the helpless poor, I have always given my advice, medicine, and exertions, with the same pleasure that I ever took the nobleman's fee, and should any other feeling possess me while I live, I should hate myself.

> "The miserable have no other medicine but only hope."

I have always thought, love to our neighbours is one of the greatest duties of human life; it constitutes the best part of our earthly happiness:

> "It is twice blessed,
> It blesseth him that gives, and him that takes;
> It is an attribute to God himself."
>   SHAKSPEARE.

I trust that my return to health will not produce in me a forgetfulness of that divine wisdom, which saw my late affliction seasonable. I was chastened. I trust I shall still go on promoting the happiness of my brethren, and consider that I am spared from death for this very end, that the remainder of my life be employed in the service of my country's good, *which is the whole world*. When all nations become united by those generous sentiments, we shall mutually encourage each other in every thing that is good. I must conclude, as I am now beyond the limits allowed me, and am still very weak, but as this may be the last opportunity I may have of addressing my fellow- creatures, I would advise them

> "To reason thus with life:
> If I do lose thee - I lose a thing
> That bearest thy heavy riches but a journey
> And death unload thee: -what's yet in this that
> Bears the name of life; lie bid more
> Thousand deaths; yet death we fear,
> That makes these odds all even." - SHAKSPEARE.

Let us consider this.

"That in the course of justice, none of us shall see salvation; we do pray for mercy, and that same prayer doth teach us all to render the deeds of mercy." - SHAKSPEARE.

May this be uppermost in the thoughts of all men, but more particularly in that of Medical men; a blessing will attend it and give them judgment to discover disease, and skill to treat it. When God endows with his favour the means which may be devised for recovering, with his assistance the humblest instrument may succeed; without it the ablest may prove unavailing. May he spare them from all sordid motives, and endow them with a spirit of pity and liberality towards the poor, and of tenderness and sympathy towards all; that they may enter into the various feelings by which they are respectively tried, may weep with those that weep, and rejoice with those that rejoice, and may he sanctify their souls as well as heal their bodies; let faith and patience, and every christian virtue they are called upon to exercise have their perfect work, so that in the end, whatever the end may be, it may be good for them to have been afflicted. Grant this, O merciful Father, through the adorable Redeemer, who while on earth went about doing good, and ever lives to make intercession for us in Heaven.

It is a reflection highly gratifying to me to know, that my practice has for a long time attracted the attention of some of the most eminent Medical men, who have acted upon the suggestion offered in former editions of this work, of personally watching the cases which have been placed either by themselves, or others, under my care; and it is with no little pride I reflect on the fact, that I am at the present time fully as much encouraged and supported by the enlightened of the profession, as by any other class of the community. It cannot be too often repeated, that these gentlemen are deserving of, and certainly have, my highest respect. There will in all cases be an independent few, breaking through the shackles of prejudice, and exhibiting that liberality and independence of mind, so creditable to human nature where it does exist. It would be a matter of surprise, in the minds of many persons, in what way my pursuits and practice have become so generally known. It may with great truth be said, that I have been sought, not that I have thrust myself on the Public. No other means have I adopted to place myself in public view, than by a small issue of several editions of this unconnected, but yet well-meaning work: and the original intention in publishing this, was rather to satisfy the inquiries, long since very generally made, than to trumpet forth my own fame.

It has been my good fortune to have been essentially useful to many leading families in this country. From a very natural wish to avoid notoriety their names never have been, (and never will by me) brought forward. But they have not been forgetful of benefits, and it is alike honourable to them, and gratifying to me, that a large portion of my patients, even in the highest stations of life, come to me, deeply prepossessed in my favour before trial - From what cause?-because some one or more of their confidential friends have so lauded my praises to them, that frequently, the greatest anxiety exists to be placed under my care (which, from my confined practice in a dwelling -house, although a large one, is often obliged to be delayed); And thus, oftentimes, through the most indirect means, I am brought into acquaintanceship with some of the most difficult cases which have yet come under my notice.

But there is another channel through which patients have reached me, which, from the frequent tone of asperity often to be found in this book against Medical Advisers, would least of all be expected —viz. through the introduction of Medical gentlemen themselves. Many of those enlightened men know and feel as I do upon the practice of medical tuition, and useless restrictions after being taught — and it is highly honourable to them as men to have acted as they have done with me. In many instances they have, first, either witnessed some portion of my practice, or taken other sure methods of ascertaining my capabilities, and then in the most liberal manner introduced me to their own patients, candidly stating that they had reason to believe I should succeed where they could not. These gentlemen cannot be too highly esteemed for thus conquering prejudices imbibed even in early youth. It cannot be matter of surprise that I should succeed, after others have failed — the reason is self - evident — the Colleges have shut out of their Pharmacopoeia some of the most useful *simples* created by the allwise Author of the universe and have constant recourse to such medicines as are of themselves frequently most injurious in their general effects, even though they may afford relief for any particular complaint. The difference is this with me, (and it is a circumstance I have repeatedly mentioned in these pages, and cannot be repeated too often), that I do not succeed by having recourse to still more violent means than have been already used (which, indeed, would in many cases be absolutely impossible); but in a large majority of cases coming under my notice, my task is two fold — first, to mitigate or remove the distressing effects of the medicine already taken; and afterwards to proceed with my own simple, harmless, and what are often called wonder-working cures. There is no mystery in this; the wonder would be if it were otherwise. Instances have repeatedly occurred of patients calling on me, at the suggestion of their own doctors, to get advice and assistance. This I am always desirous to give, under the personal observation of the Medical Adviser himself in order that he may have ocular demonstration of these things, that thus may be broken down the barrier which would prevent any one being instrumental to any useful purpose, except under the ABC tuition of the Medical Schools. It is with no little pride I reflect on the fact, that should even an attempt be made to arrest me in my useful career, among my firmest supporters would be found many of the leading Practitioners of the day, to say nothing of the nobility of the land, very many of whom are fully acquainted with my success in their own circle of relations or acquaintances.

It is with some reluctance that I have been compelled to refer to myself, both in my own remarks, and in the various letters of my patients which I have inserted. I am not aware in what way I could have explained myself sufficiently, but by so doing; as I cannot reconcile myself to printing long cases of cures performed, which might not be altogether agreeable to the parties themselves; and I am quite sure that many facts which I could have put forth, however true, would have *appeared* to border so closely on the marvellous, as to have rendered it doubtful whether they might gain belief.

I deal at all times with plainness and candour with all parties applying to me; if I see a reasonable prospect of effecting a cure, I do not hesitate a moment. At the same time I am bound to state, that many cases coming under my notice are of such long standing, and so generally relinquished as *incurable*, that it requires a considerable share of philanthropy as well as interest, to undertake them. It has been my happiness to be eminently successful, and this is reason sufficient for me to proceed, *in aid*, not in opposition to the Medical profession. Let who will, consult me, and if I can be useful to them (and this is daily occurring) I will let a *generous* rivalry exist, and I will exert every faculty I possess, before them, with them, or after them, as the case may be.

Since my illness I have had a physician from Philadelphia, in America, taking lessons from me in my mode of giving Baths and Medicine. He said he expected to have a large sum to pay me for the instruction I gave him. He expressed great surprise, on our first interview, and laying before me all his credentials from America, besides letters of introduction from the first Medical Practitioners in London, (fearing I might have a feeling of prejudice against him because he belonged to three Medical Colleges), judge of his astonishment, when I told him he should see all my apparatus, and mode of treatment, and that I was ready and willing to write him instructions and give him models of my Portable Steam Bed-Bath, the Camphor Spirit Bath; and all I could do to make him as useful in the New World, as I thought I was in the Old, and this without fee or reward. This will be the first seed of my practice sown abroad, and may a Divine Blessing attend its harvest. We have mutually exchanged many valuable receipts with each other, (this is as it ought to be: if this feeling was more general, what a happy people we should be!) . With my little Camphorated Bed-Bath he was delighted on witnessing its performance, and every medical man I have met with has pronounced it to be the most perfect, safe, and simple contrivance to obtain a copious perspiration ever offered to the public. My friends wonder I do not advertise it and take out a patent; I shall never do so, because I disapprove of the principle of an inventor paying a large sum of money to his country for having administered ease and comfort to its inhabitants. I have given liberty to my new friend to take one out in America.

I have spent more time in bringing this little apparatus into perfection, than on any other invention I ever made. No family should be without it, as by its application on the first stage of a cold, much danger and suffering might be prevented by its use; and taking one tea spoon-full of Paregoric Elixir, three ditto of Sweet Spirits of Nitre in an infusion (warm) of Elder Flowers; or it may be taken in a tumbler of warm water, sweetened with sugar. I would write one hundred more useful prescriptions for almost every disease, did I not know that as Dame Nature has made us all different in size, in complexion, in temper, in appearance , and general disposition, so we are different in our constitutions, and no one can prescribe to a certainty without an interview, or unless a patient were (which ought to be the case) conversant with his own constitution. Read Shakspeare's opinion on this subject:

> "Our heads are some brown, some black, some auburn,
> Some bald, but that our wits are so diversely coloured;
> And truly I think, if all our wits were to issue
> Out of one skull, they would fly east, west, north,
> South; and their consent of one direct way should
> Be at once to all the points o' the compass."
> SHAKSPEARE.

The habitual use of purgative medicines I have always condemned, and the many diseases arising therefrom I have often witnessed; one in particular, that of rendering the digestive organs incapable of performing their proper functions with that energy which is necessary to support the body in perfect health. I sell a new-improved portable instrument, by the use of which costiveness, and its consequences, may be always prevented. The internal parts of this little instrument being strongly coated with block tin, prevents the possibility of any metallic taint. Warm water is in most cases sufficient; but when the faeces are unusually hard, about a quarter of an ounce of white soap, dissolved in each pint of water used, will always facilitate the operation of the injection. Printed directions are given to the purchasers of this instrument with proved Recipes for

A purgative Injection,

Injection for Worms,
And Injection for Piles.

If there is any appearance of inflammation of the intestines the following emollient enema ought to be generally applied : -One pint of linseed tea or marsh -mallow tea, with two table spoon -fulls of olive oil.

There may be those who read this book that will find it difficult to get many of the herbs spoken of. To such I beg to say, although I do not profess to sell them, yet I shall feel a pleasure in accommodating persons so circumstanced, by their sending me a letter (post-paid) with a remittance; and the change (if any) will be returned with the herbs. Should my advice be required, my charge for writing a letter is 3s. 6d. to those who can afford it; when from or for the poor, I make no charge. Up to the illness before alluded to I have personally attended all my patients, and prepared my own medicines; finding I cannot continue to do so, I have prevailed on Messrs. WOOD and STEPHENSON, Practical Botanical Chemists, of No. 6, Coleman Street, City, to make extracts and liqueurs after my own manner from all the herbs spoken of on Indigestion," as they would supply me.

Parties can apply to them or me for the following: ask for the "Compound Liquor of Mountain Flax." This combines all the virtues of the herbs recommended in prescription for a foul stomach: a dessert spoonful in a little water is a dose. For a strengthening pill, ask for "The Compound Extract of Chyritaya." Those pills contain all the virtues of the strengthening herbs spoken of in Prescription 3, 4, or 5; dose 2, morning, noon, and night. I am bound in justice to say that those gentlemen have acted to my entire satisfaction;

"This will give me an estate,
Of seven years' health."
SHAKSPEARE.

(A handwritten note here states that this partnership is now dissolved, and that medicines can only be obtained from Thayer Street)

As many difficult cases of disease, not coming within the range of those to which I especially apply myself, daily present themselves, and as my time is fully occupied, with that feeling and desire to do right to which I trust that without presumption I may lay claim, I at once refuse to undertake them, and avail myself of the services of a neighbouring surgeon, one of the regulars, in whose opinion and practice I have implicit confidence. Indeed, I am bound in candour to state, that in respect to the case I have adduced of White Swelling, from Blackheath, something is due to the valuable assistance and advice which I received from this gentleman, during its progress of cure.
He is one of the few amongst the professional world who is sensibly alive to the superiority of the medicines of Nature's production over that of *art*; and has, as far as one bound in the trammels of a strictly professional education can do, availed himself of that inexhaustible store, and the vegetable extracts prepared by him for medicinal purposes are, to my own personal knowledge, genuine and effective. I am also much indebted to the valuable assistance I have received from Messrs. Sheldrake, Bigg & Co., of Leicester Square, in the ingenious contrivance of instruments for contracted knees, weak ankles, and spinal affections; in the latter I have been most successful, with my baths, suppleing the distorted parts with vegetable oils, and wearing the most peculiar and well constructed supports next the body, without the least inconvenience; they are made with that degree of niceness that relief can be given to one part while the other is compressed; this is by far more preferable and successful than the unpleasant and cruel plan of lying on the back, on a hard board, day and night, for months, and sometimes years. I have had all the credit for cures performed, but I think and feel I am bound, by that tie which constitutes that liberality of feeling which one man ought to have for another, to deal

out this meed of praise, which those gentlemen are deserving of at my hands. If the profession were thus liberal towards each other, what praise would have been due from them to that very ingenious and highly gifted man, Dr. Thornton, one of the most clever and useful botanists this country ever produced, who has for nearly thirty years been an exile from the society to which he always would have been an ornament, and for no other reason, but because his liberal practice was against the oppression practised on his fellow creatures. The cruelties he experienced so broke his spirits, that his talents have lain dormant, as a total blank, from about the year 1812 to the 22nd of January 1837, when death released him from his sufferings. For many years he has been dependent on his kind and affectionate daughters.

When his writings are once appreciated as they ought to be, and no doubt ere long will be, I should not be surprised, even in my time, to see a monument (which ought to be of gold) erected to his memory. This much ill-used man might well have said,

> "Canst thou not minister to a mind diseased,
> Pluck from the memory a rooted sorrow,
> Rase out the written troubles of the brain,
> And with some sweet oblivious antidote,
> Cleanse the bosom of that perilous stuff,
> Which weighs upon the heart?"
>
> SHAKSPEARE.

RECIPES, &c.

I shall now give a few useful receipts (sic), as proved by myself.

For an Ulcerated Sore Throat.
Half a pint of vinegar and one ounce of the herb wormwood; boil this for five minutes, and apply it warm to the throat with flannels.

For Dysentery.
One pint of vinegar, half a pound of loaf sugar, simmered in a pewter vessel, with cover of the same (no other will do). Take this quantity every day until well.

For Epileptic Fits.
One ounce of common wormwood, one ditto of mistletoe, half ditto of mountain flax; pour on this one quart of boiling water: when cold, drink a pint a day. Should there be worms, which is generally the case, this will kill and carry them off.

For a Bad Leg.
Bruise a pound of green hemlock leaves, pour on them one gallon of boiling water from a smith's forge; when cold enough, put the foot or leg into; this must be done morning and night, for twenty minutes at each time; then rasp a carrot, squeeze out the juice, warm the pulp, and fill the wound with it, cover it over with a dry rag, and confine it on with a bandage. The hemlock will not agree with some constitutions: let such apply fresh cabbage leaves, goose-grass, or clivers, bruised in the same way; at the same time take a pint a day of a strong decoction of equal parts of common mallow and clivers. Should a drying salve be required: take equal parts of unslaked lime and soap, mix well together, and dress once a day. Or with the following: - take of vinegar, resin, and myrrh, each one ounce; of red borax and ammoniac half an ounce; boil well together, and stir it until cold; this is an excellent cooling ointment if there be not much inflamation: if so, it must be first reduced by poultices.

An excellent Poultice for a Sprained or Contracted Knee.

Take equal parts of cammomile and elder flowers, bruise them in a mortar; take about the same quantity of linseed meal, mix it to a proper consistence with boiling vinegar. If there is much pain, add one ounce oil of poppies; cover the poultice with oil silk, and drink marsh mallow tea.

For a Bloated Habit similar to Dropsy.

Two ounces of foxglove boiled in a quart of water till reduced to a pint; mix this with one quart of gin, and take a wine-glass full every day for a week, and then every other day: soak the feet often, and keep then warm.

The Wild Mallow.

Whatever diversity of opinion may exist respecting the political opinions of Mr. Wm. Cobbett, none will deny his ability as a writer, or his skill as a farmer. This gentleman strongly recommends the liquor of the wild mallow for wounds. His words are:

"I cannot help mentioning here an herb which is used for medical purposes, I mean the wild mallow; it is a weed that has a leaf somwhat like a scallop, its branches spread upon the ground; it bears a seed which the children call *cheeses*, and which they string upon thread like beads. This weed is perhaps among the most valuable plants that grow; its leaves stewed, and applied wet, will cure (almost instantly cure) any cut, bruise, or wound of any sort. Poultices made of it will cure sprains, as those of the ankle; fomenting with it will remove swellings. Application of the liquor will cure the wounds caused by the friction of the saddle or collar, and its operation in all cases is so quick as hardly to be believed, it signifies not whether the wound be old or new. I gained this information upon Long Island, from a French gentleman, who was one of Buonaparte's followers in captivity. The mallows may be used directly after being gathered, merely washing off the dirt first. Like all other herbs, it should be gathered when it comes into bloom, and dried and preserved in the same manner as other herbs-it should be observed, however, that if it should happen not to be gathered at the best season, it may be gathered at any time. The root is nearly as efficacious as the branches I had two striking instances of its efficacy. A labouring farmer had cut his thumb in a dangerous manner, and after a great deal of doctoring, it was got to such a pitch, that his hand was twice the natural size; I recommended the use of the mallows, and gave him a small bunch from my store (being winter), and his hand was well in four days; he could go to work the next day, after applying the mallows oyer night. The other instance was this, I had a large and valuable hog, that had been gored by a cow; it had been in this state two days before I knew of it, and my servants looked upon it as lost; it had eaten nothing. I had it caught and held down; - the gore was in the side, and so deep that I could get my finger in beyond the ribs, - I poured in the mallows that had been stewed, and rubbed the wound with it also; the next day the hog got up and began to eat. I had him caught again, but upon examining the wound, I found it so far closed up that I did not think it right to disturb it; I had the side bathed again, and in two days he was turned out running with the others. A good handful of the herb should be boiled in a pint of water till it comes to half a pint. Now a person must be almost criminally careless not to make provision of this herb."

This is one of my most useful herbs, and many wounds that I have cured with its assistance, have fully equalled what here is stated. I have given it successfully for the gravel; and to persons of a costive habit of body, I believe nothing can surpass it; if it be taken every day for a month, in a decoction for infusion, it will, from its oily nature, entirely do away with the necessity of *forcing* medicines, which generally do more harm than good. When the bowels do not perform their functions with regularity, there will infallibly arise consequences more or less destructive to health. I strongly recommend the following Prescription:

> Two ounces of dried Marsh Mallows,
> One ounce of Parsley Root,
> Two drachms of Mountain Flax.

Boil this in one quart of water till reduced to one pint, drink this in the course of the day; the action of this decoction is more of a diuretic than a carthatic nature, by which much of that slimy matter which corrodes the kidneys is carried off. I wish strongly to impress on the minds of my readers, (and I speak from experience), that more depends on a pure and proper state of the secretions of those organs, than any other function carried on in the body. Every alternate day drink about a pint of the following decoction:

> Four ounces of Sarsaparilla sliced,
> One ounce of Sassafras sliced,
> One ounce of Guiacum Wood,
> Two ounces of Liquorice Root bruised,
> Half an ounce of Mezereon Root;

the sarsaparilla ought to be first boiled by itself in three quarts of water until reduced to two quarts, then add the other ingredients and boil for half an hour.

To prevent Sea Sickness.

> One ounce of Opium,
> Two drachms Extract of Henbane,
> Ten grains of powdered Mace,
> Two ounces of hard Mottled Soap;

boil this in three pints of water for half an hour, stirring it all the time; when cold, add one quart of spirits of wine, and two drachms of spirit of ammonia. Rub a table-spoonful of this embrocation all over the stomach, and particularly over the breast-bone and under the left ribs, for several days before embarkation. This quantity must be rubbed in two or three times a day for the first part of the voyage, until sickness ceases. The bowels ought to be kept active with salts and senna the last week or fortnight on shore, but in most constitutions the rubbing alone is sufficient.

For the Tooth-Ache.

Take two parts of the leaves of rue, and one part salt; form this into little balls, and place one in the hollow of the ear on the side opposite to that of the aching tooth; this produces a great warmth, and in most cases relieves the pain.

Another.

Take a lump of unslacked lime the size of a walnut; put it into three parts of a tumbler of cold water; when cold enough, hold it in the mouth, on the painful tooth: let this be repeated as often as the pain is felt.

I recommend the following infusion to be freely drank by all persons while taking my Gout and Family Pills, either as a cure or a preventative.

Take liquorice root, coltsfoot, elder flowers, holy thistle, juniper berries bruised, and green sage, of each one ounce; placing them in a jug, add two quarts of boiling water, stop it down close and let it stand near the fire for three hours to simmer (not to boil, as that will pass off the essential oil of herbs by evaporation), then strain for use.

These few simple Receipts (sic) will be found useful in many private families. Since my last work was published, I have frequently had persons apply to me from a great distance with my book in their hands. I have opened it on hearing their case, and shown them, if they had attended to my printed advice, they might have spared themselves the trouble and expense of coming to me. The answer generally is, "Bless me, Sir, I never noticed that;" or "I was afraid to try it until I had seen you." -I have sent such away empty-handed to try my remedies, which perhaps for a cure may cost them one shilling and six pence. I have many letters, thanking me for this (what they please to call generous) act, and informing me that they have not only cured themselves, but their poor neighbours. These reports always give me great pleasure, as my great aim has, and I trust ever will be, to instruct others, not to enrichen myself by their misfortunes.

I wish now to draw my readers' attention to this my last Hint, which is of as much or more importance than any I have before given. To persons who suffer from nervous head-ache and indigestion, (and who is there that does not, who have had their constitutions abused by the use of mercury), to such I would refer to a remark in a former page, of keeping their feet SWEET and CLEAN, and plenty of room in the shoe for the blood to circulate in all the small beautiful veins of the toes, which cannot be the case if the foot is contracted, when it becomes cold and numbed. That gentle perspiration of the body which ought to keep the feet in a glow of moisture to throw off the dross of the humours as they descend, ascends to the head, and causes those painful sensations so much felt by both sexes, but more so by females, as they bear the additional evil of having their body in a *vice*, commonly called stays. Now the merely sponging or washing the feet is not sufficient; they ought, once or twice a week, to be well soaked in hot water, then take a thick piece of flannel, such as ironing blanket, and lather it well with one part soap and one part pipe clay, this application will get out all the dandriff, scurf, or dead skin, and leave the pores open; then there would be no disagreeable smell, as is too often the case when the humours are shut in by a false skin formed all over the feet. All my readers must have felt (or seen in others), that when there is this burning heat in the feet instead of the warmth produced by perspiration, that they swell by day, but on the following morning are reduced to their natural size; this is easily accounted for, as when the body is laid flat in bed those humours drain back into the system, and impregnate all the healthy parts of the body. Such persons will be found more cheerful towards the close of the day, as those humours (which are like the lees of beer or wine) fall down; but in the morning feel sick and low spirited, with a disrelish for food or exercise, and, in fact, disagreeable to themselves and all around them; and all this may arise from not being particular with their feet, which carry all the burthen, as they are with their hands and face. I may be wrong in this opinion, yet

"This still may help to thicken other proofs
That do demonstrate thinly."
SHAKSPEARE.

It is by attending to such simples as these that I ascribe my success in curing and preventing disease; besides I am only following the directions of *Nature's child*, who advises,

"By telling me the sovereign'st thing on earth
Was spermaceti for an inward bruise,"
SHAKSPEARE.

In an earlier page of this book, one of my patients in his letter, speaks of the establishment of a Hospital for the more extended adoption of my practice, as one mode of enabling me to be more extensively use my fellow creatures, than I am now individually enabled to do, without assistance of any description. I should rejoice in the realization of this project, which, indeed, is not a new proposition, for had the late Lord Robert Seymour been spared a few years longer, it was determined by him to be carried into effect- either by his own purse, or with the assistance of others possessing the same charitable feeling as this most excellent nobleman. (This most excellent Nobleman spent large sums in relieving the distresses of the poor; and it was my privilege to be his almoner for many years. When real distress has been pointed to him, he would not sleep till I had visited it,—and often I have gone, even at midnight, to report to him the particulars of some case in which he has been deeply interested, and found him waiting patiently for my arrival. His honoured widow continues in the same path; and very recently I have received a sum from her Ladyship, for the relief of a fatherless family, reduced from affluence to beggary. "Verily they have their reward!")

And who can doubt, that the persevering efforts of the same christian zeal which succeeded in the founding of the splendid Lunatic establishment at Hanwell, would have likewise succeeded in opening a building, where the practice which I have long been carrying on in my own house, might have been more extensively adopted, by the assistance of well selected students, whose academical knowledge, blended with my useful practice, would succeed in convincing the world, that no good reason exists, why the Royal College of Surgeons should not pursue *their* path, and I proceed in the even tenor of *my way*, and a few months would enable the public to know, what is already most extensively known to many noble families and talented individuals of this land, including many first-rate practitioners, that I have, first, the ability to be most extensively useful to my fellow creatures; and secondly, that I am not wanting in those feelings which would induce any man, having received gifts from God, to use them for the benefit of mankind.

Life is uncertain-the number of my days is equally uncertain. Should not, therefore, some effort be made to perpetuate my system, which is known to hundreds as being a great blessing to all who have recourse to it? I have advised previously that plenty of room should be allowed in the shoe, for the blood to circulate freely. For this purpose I recommend

HALL & Co.'s PANNUS- CORIUM,
or LEATHER- CLOTH BOOTS AND SHOES,

sold by the Patentees, Wellington Street, Waterloo Bridge, Strand. I constantly wear them, and think them most excellent for the purpose intended.

Ease and Comfort in Walking, Softness and Elasticity to the most sensitive parts of the feet, combined with the durability and appearance of ordinary Leather, are the leading features and re commendations of this invention.

It will be seen by the following extract from their Testimonials, that their invention has received Royal Patronage.

Extract of a letter from THEIR MAJESTIES, through SIR HERBERT TAYLOR, K.C.B. , G.C.H.

Windsor Castle, June 4th, 1831.

GENTLEMEN,

Having submitted your Letter of May 28th, with the accompanying specimens of Patent Pannus Corium , or Leather-Cloth Shoes, to Their Majesties, I am honoured with Their commands to acquaint you with Their approval of them.

I am, Gentlemen,
Your obedient Servant,
H, TAYLOR.

To Messrs. Hall & Co. 109, Strand.

Sir Herbert Taylor begs to acknowledge the receipt of Messrs. Halls' Letter of the 18th instant, and to acquaint them, that his Majesty has no objection to their styling themselves "Leather Cloth Boot and Shoe Makers to his Majesty." Those made for Sir Herbert answer extremely well, and he will recommend them generally.

Windsor Castle, August 20th, 1831,

TILKE'S

CAMPHORATED SPIRIT LAMP,

FOR

GIVING A BED BATH.

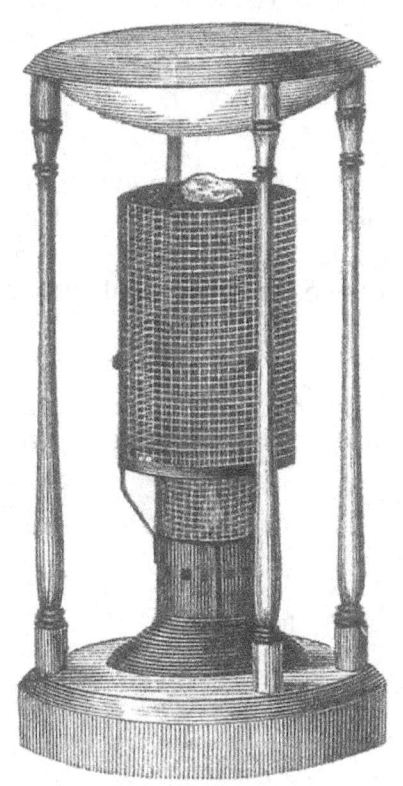

From a Drawing by Miss J. W. Tilke.

Directions for Using the Camphorated Spirit Lamp.

Take off the wire, unscrew the burner, and put one ounce of spirits of wine into the receiver; screw on again, set light, and fix on the wire, on the top of which put about one ounce of camphor; this, with the wick of the length herewith sent (and it never ought to be higher) will burn one hour. It may be placed in bed, by the side of the patient, where the disease is acute, as in Rheumatism, &c. It is surprisingly efficacious in Influenza, Cholera, violent Colds, &c. A very thick covering of bed-clothes is required to keep the heat in. As a domestic comfort, this little apparatus is invaluable, portable, simple, and easily used without assistance. Beds may be warmed and aired by it. To enumerate the various diseases that may be cured by profuse perspiration would be superfluous. For general use, the patient is required to lay on his back, the lamp being placed between the knees; the sticks sent with the lamp are to be used, one on each side, to support the bed-clothes, which must be well tucked in round the neck. There should at no time be more spirit put in the lamp than is intended for present use; should any be left for a few days in the reservoir, it acts on the tin and causes rust; the spirit also evaporates, which leaves the wick wet, and on the next occasion it will not burn. If the spirit is all consumed, one wick will last for twelve months.

Extract from a letter written by a medical gentleman, who employs it in his practice with the most pleasing results:

"The more I witness the good effects of your extraordinary and clever little Camphorated Bath, the more I am surprised that you do not make its usefulness known, by advertisements, at this moment, when the prevailing disease of Influenza is sweeping away thousands from the land; its use is invaluable. I am sure no person, medical or non medical, would be without one if they were once to know its value."

This Bath is very serviceable to persons subject to Gout, as the use of it, when symptoms of Gout are felt, will effectually keep it off-and, *with* the Gout, it is found very active in bringing relief, taking at the same time the following:

One tea-spoon full of Paregoric Elixir,
Three ditto Sweet Spirits of Nitre,
in an infusion (warm) of Elder Flower.

SOLD ONLY BY THE INVENTOR,

Price Thirty-five Shillings,

At No. 8, Thayer -Street, Manchester -Square.

Published Previously.

OBSERVATIONS

ON

THE NATURE OF GOUT,

RING - WORM,

AND

SCARLET FEVER.

By S. W. TILKE.

1834